"Yoga has benefited the lives of people for millennia. Its power to promote human health has now been verified scientifically. In this book, Suza Francina shows how anyone can reap the healing benefits of this ancient yet modern therapy."

Larry Dossey, M.D.
author, *Be Careful What You Pray For, Prayer Is Good Medicine* and *Healing Words*
executive editor, *Alternative Therapies in Health and Medicine*

"Few people are as qualified as Suza Francina to write about the life-enhancing benefits of yoga for those over 50. Ms. Francina's book confirms my own experience as well as inspires me to continue yoga with enthusiasm and confidence. What better gift can we give ourselves than the ability to move, breath and enjoy life, whatever our age."

Judith H. Lasater, Ph.D.
physical therapist, author, *Relax & Renew: Restful Yoga for Stressful Times*

"This is the book we've been waiting for! At last, we latecomers to yoga have a commonsense guide that initiates us in a way that is eminently "do-able." We're recommending it to our patients as a means of freeing both mind and body from the inner tension and outward rigidity that foster anxiety and depression."

John E. Nelson, M.D., and Andrea Nelson, Psy.D.
editors, *Sacred Sorrows, Embracing and Transforming Depression*

"The *New Yoga for People Over 50* will be my constant companion. In this crazy world that loves control, where most people are trying desperately just to cope, *The New Yoga for People Over 50* gives me the energy and flexibility to swim the laps, work at home and in the garden, be a grandma and laugh with my friends and family."

Malchia Olshan
swim champion, National Masters and Senior Olympics

"Studying with Vanda Scaravelli through her late 70s and 80s gave me a remarkable vision of aging. I hope Suza Francina's new book, filled with success stories about older teachers and students, will inspire many people of all ages to embark on the wonderful path of growth and transformation we call yoga."

Esther Myers
author, *Yoga and You: Energizing and Relaxing Yoga for New and Experienced Students*

"Master Iyengar yoga instructor Suza Francina has distilled a lifetime of teaching into a practical handbook that anyone can use to improve their health. I've strengthened my back muscles and increased my flexibility using her methods. I recommend this book to all, especially those who want to improve the quality of their life and health in midlife and beyond."

George Jaidar
author, *The Soul: An Owner's Manual, Discovering the Life of Fullness*

"I loved the people in this book! Their stories show how yoga can expand an older person's world, help them to improve their posture and health and bring them joy. They are an inspiration."

Noreen Morris, R.N., S.C.M.
hospice nurse and yoga student

"*The New Yoga for People Over 50* presents delightful vignettes of real people who have used yoga to improve the quality of their lives. I wholeheartedly agree with Suza Francina that youthfulness, strength and flexibility are not prerequisites to yoga practice, but are its benefits. Most important, her book makes them available to students of all ages."

Mary Pullig Schatz, M.D.
author, *Back Care Basics: A Doctor's Gentle Yoga Program for Back and Neck Pain Relief*

"After dedicating myself to walking for health, fitness and peace of mind for over twelve years, I realized in my mid-forties that it simply was not enough. My body had aches and pains and stiffness, and I knew I needed to pay attention to stretching. Suza's book came into my life when I needed the inspiration of stories of people much older than me who were more flexible and dynamic physically than I was when I was twenty!"

Maggie Spilner
walking editor, *Prevention Magazine*
coauthor, *Prevention's Practical Encyclopedia of Walking for Health*

"Suza Francina presents yoga in an intelligent, dignified and accessible form. I recommend her new book to anyone interested in health, vigor and quality of life."

Dean Ornish, M.D.
author, *Dr. Dean Ornish's Program for Reversing Heart Disease*

"I began studying yoga at 50. In a year it changed the shape of my body and flexibility of my spine. I now recommend yoga to all my patients. People over 50 often say they expect to have aches and pains. *The New Yoga for People Over 50* dispels that myth! Patients who are practicing yoga are rarely in acute back pain. Their adjustments hold longer. Yoga really enhances chiropractic care."

Jane Chalmers, D.C., F. I. A. C. A.

"Having just read Suza Francina's book, I felt yoga might be a good place to start my quest for a lifestyle that would allow me to be independent as long as possible. So at the age of 72, and having just lost my beloved husband of 49 years, I tried yoga for the first time in my life. That decision turned out to be one of the best I've ever made. The physical effort, the weight-bearing exercise, the feeling of accomplishment combined to give me a tremendous boost in self-esteem. This book helped point me in the direction I want to go!"

Helen McKeown
72-year-old yoga student

"This book offers a wealth of information to help alleviate the problems associated with aging. The stories from older practitioners and teachers B.K.S. Iyengar, Indra Devi and Eric Small are especially uplifting and inspiring."

Donald Moyer
director, The Yoga Room, Berkeley, California

The New Yoga for People Over 50

A Comprehensive Guide for Midlife and Older Beginners

Suza Francina

Health Communications, Inc.
Deerfield Beach, Florida

www.hci-online.com

We would like to acknowledge the publishers and individuals below for permission to reprint the following material:

Photographs on pages xix, 1, 8, 9, 12, 15, 30, 35, 36, 37, 40, 41, 43, 47, 55, 57, 69, 71, 75, 76, 79, 80, 86, 102, 104, 109, 125, 133, 151, 172, 174, 176, 177, 211, 215, 221, 227, 231, 234 and 235 reprinted with permission of Jim Jacobs. ©1997 Jim Jacobs.

Photographs on pages 54, 122, 123, 128, 129, 135, 138, 140, 143, 144 and 246 reprinted with permission of Paul Del Signore Photography. ©1996 Paul Del Signore.

Photographs on pages vii, 22 and 216 reprinted with permission of John Henebry. ©1997 John Henebry.

Photographs on pages xvii, xxii, xxvii, 17, 29, 38, 45, 49, 52, 66, 68, 72, 73, 101, 170, 171 and 222 reprinted with permission of Ron Seba. ©1993 Ron Seba.

Photographs on pages xxvii, 64 and 238 reprinted with permission of Benette Rottman. ©1993 Benette Rottman.

Photograph on page 207 reprinted with permission of Nils Larsen. ©1993 Nils Larsen.

(Continued on page 281)

Library of Congress Cataloging-in-Publication Data

Francina, Suza, (date)
    The new yoga for people over 50: a comprehensive guide for midlife and older beginners / Suza Francina.
      p. cm.
    Includes bibliographical references.
    ISBN 1-55874-453-3 (pbk.: alk. paper)
    1. Yoga, Hatha. 2. Middle aged persons—Health and hygiene. 3. Aged—Health and hygiene. I. Title.
RA781.7.F7 1997   97-20984
613.7'046—dc21   CIP

©1997 Suza Francina
ISBN 1-55874-453-3

Publisher: Health Communications, Inc.
           3201 S.W. 15th Street
           Deerfield Beach, Florida 33442-8190

Cover design by Andrea Perrine Brower
Cover photo of Betty Eiler by Jim Jacobs

For my students
at the Ojai Yoga Center
and my children,
Bo and Monica Hebenstreit

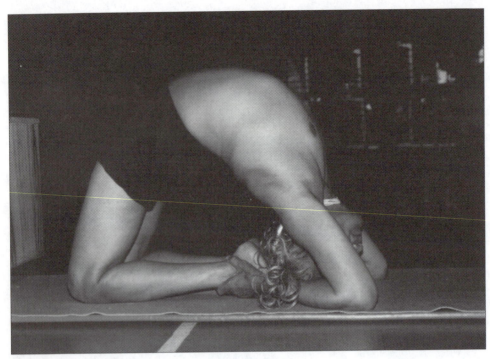

B.K.S. Iyengar at age 75.

Yoga is an immortal art, science and philosophy.
It is the best subjective psycho-anatomy of mankind ever
conceived for the experience of physical, mental, intellectual, and
spiritual well-being. It has stood the test of time from the
beginning of civilization and it will remain supreme as a precise
psycho-physical science for centuries to come.

—B.K.S. Iyengar, author of *Light on Yoga,*
Light on Pranayama and other treatises on yoga.
Born on December 14, 1918, Iyengar still performs a
rigorous daily yoga practice that would challenge
anyone at any age.

Contents

Foreword

⁓

With today's technological advances and health consciousness, I do not consider those over fifty to be old. However, in many cases, people above sixty allow their bodies and minds to sink into declining wavelengths of energy and thought.

One has to accept changes in body function as a natural part of the life cycle. When nature perceives weakness in a person's thinking, it contracts and shrinks the cellular system, affecting the supply of blood and bio-energy. This decline in blood and bio-energy dries the psychological spheres as well, creating dullness in oneself and, at times, a negative attitude toward life.

However, it is the duty of the aging person both to accept the game that nature plays, and to resist it by activating the "willpower"—the sharp blade of mind and intelligence. By using willpower, one can arrest the deteriorating process and develop the constituents of health (respiratory, circulatory and bio-energetic systems) to an optimum level.

Health is like a live wire—very sensitive. Health flows like a river ever refreshing and alive. Health is not like a stagnant pool. So attention to the body and mind should be of the highest voltage of intelligence. Truly, as people age, taking care of the body should be a priority.

Daily practice of yoga will keep old age at bay. Yoga transforms a negative approach to life into a positive dynamic one. It helps us to take care of ourselves at times of need. Practicing yoga also brings into play the body's natural ability to arrest the deteriorating process. It enables us to endure what cannot be cured and makes the entire cycle of life worth living.

Be aware that while young people have powerful bodies, they need the disciplines of ethics and philosophy. Older people, like myself, have the discipline and, hence, are fit to start yoga (if they have not begun it already) so that the chariot (the body) and the charioteer (the Self) live together with contentment and bliss. Only good, caring guidance is necessary to help aging people achieve this.

Suza Francina presents yoga in a way that creates confidence in readers to be independent and strong.

I, at eighty proudly invite you, my fellow human beings, to take a dip into yoga. I was afflicted with tuberculosis when I was thirteen. I took to yoga to taste the nectar of health. Even at this age I practice yoga with zeal for four to five hours a day, keeping myself young in body, mind and Soul.

I am writing this in the spirit of love for members of my age group, to encourage them to pay attention to their bodies so that they remain their true friends in times of need.

Yours faithfully,

B.K.S. Iyengar
Ramamani Iyengar Memorial Yoga Institute Shivajinagar
March 16, 1998

Acknowledgments

⁓

First and foremost I wish to thank my students in the Yoga-Over-60 program at the Ojai Yoga Center, my living laboratory. Their sense of adventure and growth inspires me daily. I am also grateful to the students and teachers from all over the world who responded to my questionnaire and shared their stories, interviews and photographs. Their letters of support and proddings about when the book would be done have helped me to persevere. My special thanks go to Betty Eiler and her students for their enthusiastic contributions.

I also want to thank my partner at the Ojai Yoga Center, Judi Flannery-Lukas, who taught for me endlessly so I could finish this manuscript. Judi's trips to India to study at the Ramamani Iyengar Memorial Institute have illuminated our Yoga Center with "Light on Yoga."

Likewise, I want to express my appreciation to the teachers at The Iyengar Yoga Institute in San Francisco and to other teachers I have studied with over the years, especially Diana Clifton and Felicity Green. You opened my eyes and dispelled all my notions about aging, both by your personal example and the confidence with which you took students more than twice my age into Handstands at a time when this pose put the fear of God into me.

Thanks to B.K.S. Iyengar for permission to use his photos and quotes on yoga, health and aging. I was almost as impressed by his prompt response to my inquiry (living proof that he does not procrastinate like the rest of us mortals!) as I was with his inspiring demonstration of the yoga poses at age 75 during his visit to the U.S.

I hardly know how to thank photographer Jim Jacobs who appeared on the horizon at exactly the right moment. A serious yoga-over-50 practitioner himself, Jim has a special passion for photographing older people exhibiting beauty, grace and character. The photographs of his teacher, Ramanand Patel, and others enliven the pages of this book.

And then there are the many people who have helped me directly and indirectly over the years to complete this project—my agent, Barbara Neighbors Deal, for bringing the manuscript to the attention of my publisher; Karen Marita, for secretarial assistance and keeping my house and family afloat; Malchia Olshan and George Jaidar, surrogate parents who dried my tears and helped me to grow up; Barbara Uniker, Michael Callahan, Lyn Hebenstreit, Dale Hanson, Robert Houston, Chip Lukas, George and Jean Kalogridis, Julie Cross Hebenstreit and my parents, Mary and René Diets, for their invaluable support.

Thank you also, Judith Gustafson, for casting light on my computer, searching out typos and extra spaces, and for endless hours of all kinds of help. I deeply appreciate your friendship through thick and thin, for better and for worse.

I want to express my appreciation to everyone at Health Communications Inc., who helped assure that this book would see the light of day. Peter Vegso and Gary Seidler, HCI's president and vice president and avid yoga students, for believing in the project. Christine Belleris for discovering this book in her mountain of prospective manuscripts and guiding it through the editorial process. Andrea Perrine Brower for her cover design. Lawna Oldfield, for the text layout and design. And the rest of the talented HCI staff: Allison Janse, Kim Weiss, Ronni O'Brien, Kelly Johnson Maragni, Kathryn Butterfield and Randee Goldsmith.

Last, but not least, Karen McAuley, the Mr. Iyengar of editors—merciless, rigorous, unrelenting. Every day for many months as I sat chained bleary-eyed to the computer, pecking away with one hopeless finger, she would arrive on her bicycle, take one cheerful look at my rambling efforts, and insist then and there that I streamline and clarify my thoughts. Her daily presence as she scrutinized each page has been both a curse and a blessing. This book has been a true test of our friendship.

Introduction

Welcome to the New Yoga for People Over 50!

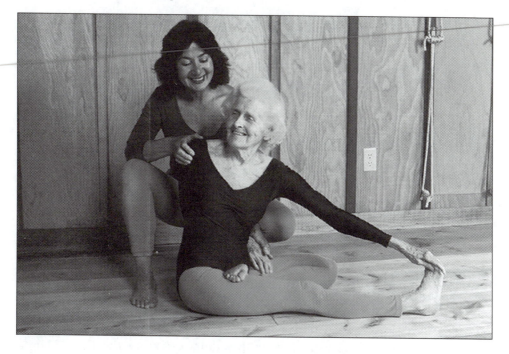

Yoga is a gift for older people. One who studies yoga in the later years gains not only health and happiness, but also freshness of mind since yoga gives one a bright outlook on life. One can look forward to a satisfying, more healthful future rather than looking back into the past. With yoga, a new life begins, even if started later. Yoga is a rebirth which teaches one to face the rest of one's life happily, peacefully and courageously.

—Geeta S. Iyengar, *Yoga, A Gem for Women*

As preventive medicine,
yoga is unequaled.

—KAREEM ABDUL-JABBAR

Twenty years have passed since I wrote the first edition of *Yoga for People Over 50.* The time has gone by in the twinkling of an eye, and many of my students who began yoga after age 60 are now in their 80s. Recently, when one of my octogenarians remarked how challenging the "Over-60 Class" was for newcomers, they laughingly decided to call themselves the "Advanced Old Age Class." The members of this class are the most dedicated and have the best attendance record of all my students because, they've told me, "We don't dare miss! We don't dare quit!"

When new students drop in on the class, thinking it's going to be easy, the experienced students seem to get a thrill out of staying in Downward-Facing Dog long after the gaping novice collapses. The octogenarians especially enjoy demonstrating the Right-Angle Handstand, a pose requiring upper-body strength, flexibility and a little bit of daring. It's all in good fun, of course, and generally inspires new people to start practicing.

You are as young as
your spine is flexible.
—*Source Unknown*

I see the biggest changes among my students who come regularly two or three times a week for several years. It is a source of inspiration and encouragement to see someone over 60 practicing poses that people of any age may find difficult when starting out. I know how impressed I was by my teachers who were more than 40 years older and far more supple than I was.

It's one thing to be under 20 and practicing all these wonderful, exotic-looking poses, and people can just shrug and say, "Well, she's still young. Her body can do that naturally." But when you see older students and teachers practicing difficult poses with relative ease, poses that your poor stiff body perhaps half their age can only dream about, then you start to wake up and realize that *yoga really works!*

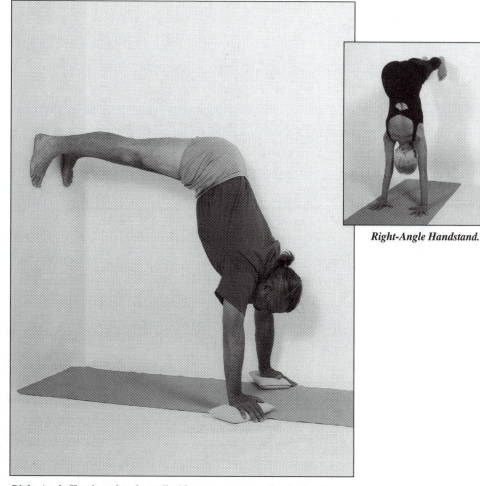

Right-Angle Handstand.

Right-Angle Handstand at the wall with extra support under the hands.

At every stage of
spiritual growth, the
greatest ally you
have is your body.

—*Deepak Chopra, M.D.,*
Ageless Body, Timeless
Mind: The Quantum
Alternative to Growing Old

You're never too old to do yoga. On the contrary, you're too old *not* to do yoga! No segment of our population can benefit more from yoga than people over 50. In fact, the older you are, the more you will benefit from practicing this ancient science and healing art. Yoga goes against the grain by removing the stiffness and inertia from the body. "It takes time to take care of your self," I remind my students, "but it takes even more time if you don't take care of your self." Yoga improves the quality of life for people of all ages, but most especially for those who are older.

My teaching experience confirms what Dr. Deepak Chopra and other experts on aging have written: that older people in particular need a conscious, non-mechanical, intelligent, expansive approach to exercise that involves the whole person—body, mind and spirit. The fragmented geriatric exercise and rehabilitation programs commonly prescribed are of limited benefit to seniors. Yoga's preventive and rehabilitative gifts are becoming more widely known; even more important is yoga's timeless wisdom that aging can bring greater perspective and illumination, expanded awareness and continuing growth, rather than deterioration. This underlying philosophy can help an aging population bring balance to our culture's obsession with the super-ficial trappings of youth.

How I Began Teaching Yoga

Like many of my generation, I began practicing yoga from books in the late 1960s and early 1970s. My first teachers were older men and women who were considered, back then, eccentric senior citizen types—

that is, they were pioneers far ahead of their time. In the first edition of my book, published in 1977, I described the pleasant agony my body experienced while attempting to mimic instructors more than twice my age. During the first yoga class I ever attended, I was situated between two students in their mid-60s. They were bending and stretching like youngsters while I, not half their age, felt as if my poor, stiff back was stuck in cement. I didn't feel too kindly toward the flexible 60-year-old teacher who told me outright that "if we grow old and stiff, we have no one to blame but ourselves."

While I was starting yoga, I was working as a home health-care provider for convalescents and the elderly, something I had done since my teens. I befriended and cared for many of these same people until they died, some of them for as long as 25 years. This gave me the opportunity to observe firsthand the mental and physical changes that often occur in the later years. The contrast between the elderly people I cared for and the seemingly ageless yoga practitioners I met was striking. The people who practiced yoga showed almost no evidence of such common problems as arthritis, bone fractures caused by osteoporosis, heart conditions, breathing problems, incontinence, confusion, memory loss and other problems mistakenly blamed on aging.

When I first began teaching yoga at a local senior center, like most young, enthusiastic but ignorant exercise instructors, I thought that older people were very stiff and brittle and that they would break if I asked them to bend. I automatically relegated people with white hair to armchair exercises or gentle stretches on the floor. Gradually, as I gained experience and confidence, I saw that as with

> Yoga is for everyone, at any age. You can begin at any time of your life. If you are over 65 and an absolute beginner, welcome! There is no better time to start than this moment!
> —Lilias Folan, author of Lilias, Yoga and Your Life

any age group, older people come into a yoga class with various levels of ability and medical histories.

While both the frail elderly and late-life yoga students with severe balance problems may initially benefit and gain confidence by practicing modified yoga postures sitting in a chair, practicing in this way can be counterproductive to the goal of keeping older students independent and out of a wheelchair. In 20 years of teaching yoga to older beginners, I've learned that most

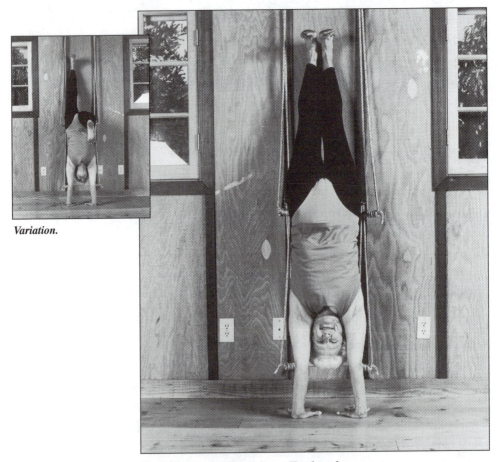

Variation.

Sandy Yost, in her 70s, enjoys a Handstand.

can benefit from the same vital weight-bearing postures that are taught in my regular classes, while those with medical problems such as heart disease, high blood pressure, osteoporosis, arthritis and other concerns discussed in this book can practice at a slower pace and with modified poses.

People of all ages generally start yoga to stretch the "kinks" out of their body, to strengthen their bones and muscles, to improve their posture, to breathe better, to relax and improve their overall health and vitality. Older students who attend class regularly for at least six months report that their increased strength and range of movement enables them to return to physical activities they thought they had lost forever: gardening, climbing uphill or climbing stairs, biking, dancing, reaching and bending without strain, being able to sit comfortably on the floor in various positions, and getting up and off the floor with confidence.

My older students and teachers are pioneers—positive role models who demonstrate that yoga reverses the aging process and allows us to enjoy our bodies well into our real old age.

What You Will Find in This Book

Throughout this book you will find inspiring photographs, quotes and personal stories of teachers and students from all over the world, many in their 70s and older, who demonstrate that age is irrelevant when it comes to practicing and enjoying the benefits of yoga. B.K.S. Iyengar, born in 1918, still performs a rigorous daily yoga practice. Also featured are Diana Clifton, a highly respected teacher in her mid-70s; Vanda Scaravelli, born in 1908, and author of *Awakening the Spine;* and Indra Devi, who, when I interviewed her at age 94, was still traveling the world, lecturing on the benefits of yoga. Many other practitioners who began yoga after midlife, and who overcame various health problems associated with aging, appear throughout the text.

The beginning chapters of this book explore the changing view of aging and yoga's well-known reputation for slowing down and reversing the premature aging process. You will learn how the health of your spine and posture affects every system of the body and how yoga postures and breathing exercises affect the circulatory system, the heart and other vital organs. Physicians and physiologists have long recognized that reversing gravity, by inverting parts or all of the body, has a beneficial effect on the circulation, lungs and brain. After 50 it becomes increasingly important to reverse the downward pull of gravity, and the benefits and precautions of turning the body halfway and completely upside down are explained.

The New Yoga for People Over 50 also explores yoga's special benefits for women during the menopausal years, how yoga strengthens our bones and helps prevent osteoporosis and arthritis, yoga's role in preventing and reversing heart disease, and other common health concerns of those of us at midlife and older.

The practice guides that appear throughout the book demonstrate how yoga props—bolsters, straps, chairs, backbending benches, walls and wall ropes—enable older students to experience the benefits of difficult or challenging poses safely. Yoga props help teach the principles of correct body alignment and correct movement, and work to improve strength, flexibility, balance and endurance. Props also provide support for the practice of many deeply relaxing, rejuvenating, restorative postures.

The practice guides focus on the special needs of middle-aged and older people who have begun to feel the "wearing down" effect of other forms of exercise, or who may be coming to yoga with various health problems. Directions are geared to beginners well over 50 and demonstrate how the more challenging yoga postures, which are whole-body movements, can more easily be learned in their component parts. In the beginning, many of the more difficult positions can be practiced lying on the floor or with the support of a wall or chair, and stretching each part of the body individually, removing the stiffness from the body one joint at a time.

Despite the fact that people over 50 can be in better physical condition than those half their age, professionally prescribed home exercise routines, specifically designed for the "geriatric adult" or "geriatric segment of the population," still tend to relegate the older practitioner to easy generic exercises done on the floor, in a chair or wheelchair, bed or bathtub. This book describes and illustrates how older beginners can adapt the practice of yoga to their special needs, including medical considerations such as cardiovascular disease, arthritis, hip surgery and osteoporosis, and also how they can safely progress.

The practice guides were tested in class on students who started practicing yoga after the age of 70, 80 and older, and demonstrate how even those beginners with difficulty getting up from the floor can progress from gentle floor and chair stretching to vital weight-bearing standing and inverted postures. Beginners will gain confidence practicing at home and in a class setting.

Use Common Sense!

My purpose in featuring older yoga practitioners is to encourage readers of all ages to exercise in a way that will keep their bodies healthy for a lifetime. I wish to remind readers that the more advanced postures, all demonstrated by people well over 50, are best learned under the guidance of an experienced and qualified instructor.

I especially want to caution readers not to strain their knees by attempting prematurely to sit in the Lotus posture or other more advanced bent-knee seated positions. Over the years, many overzealous Westerners have learned the hard way that the knee is a most unforgiving joint. If your knees have become stiff from years of sitting in a chair, refer to the practice guides in chapters 3, 5 and 8 for safe stretches to remove the stiffness from your hips and knees.

The directions for practicing yoga in this book are based on an approach developed by one of the most influential yoga teachers of this century, B.K.S. Iyengar. Iyengar yoga is known for its emphasis on developing strength, flexibility, endurance and correct body alignment. Standing poses unique to Iyengar yoga strengthen the whole body and are known to relieve many common back and neck problems. They also help to correct foot, ankle and knee problems, which are almost epidemic in our culture in the over-50 population. You will find further information in chapter 5 on yoga for feet and knees.

I hope that this book will bring yoga to the attention of those who are ready to reject the notion that aging is a process of decline and who will encourage many other people to explore yoga's ascending path to physical and spiritual transformation.

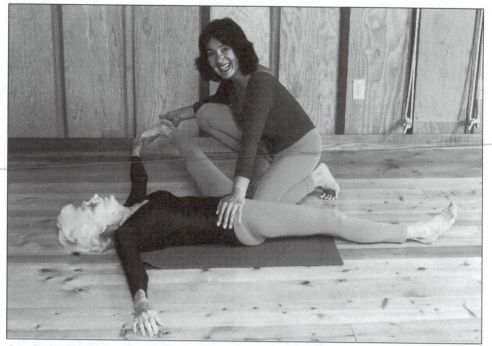

Suza Francina helps a student stretch her legs.

No book can ever replace a teacher who directs, adjusts, encourages and inspires you. It is my dream that *The New Yoga for People Over 50* will motivate many more people to attend their local yoga classes.

Frank White:
Yoga, A Better Way to Spend the
Autumn and Winter Years

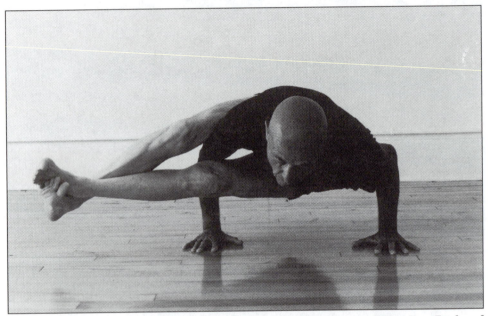

Frank White, 76, demonstrates an advanced balance pose. He was honored in 1993 as Yoga Teacher of the Year.

I am in better shape now than when I was 40. I can move better. I'm more flexible. I'm stronger, with more stamina. Yoga absolutely not only retards, but reverses the aging process.

I was in my 66th year of life, and it was becoming increasingly difficult to get out of bed in the morning. Stiffness and pain in my spine, legs and joints were keeping me from doing all the wonderful things that my body was capable of doing as a younger person. Something was gradually taking away my freedom of movement.

The doctors called it "severe degenerative osteoarthritis"— a very fancy name for a crippling disease. I just called it "plain misery." Depressed and anxious, the spark and zest for life that I once had were rapidly diminishing.

I had been under the care of a cardiologist for about 15 years for hypertensive cardiovascular disease (high blood pressure) and arteriosclerosis. I took medication daily. Not a pleasant way to spend the autumn and winter years of my life.

Somehow I found myself in a yoga class. Not only did I know that I was home, but I realized that a miraculous, almost magical transformation was possible. When I finished the class, I was weeping. Something released inside my body that said, "YES!"

From that day until the present—and I am now 76 years old—I have been doing yoga on a daily basis. I became a vegetarian and, as my life transformed, so did my health. I lost 50 pounds. My blood pressure returned to normal without medication. My cholesterol dropped from 400 to 150.

I became a yoga instructor and am devoting my life to teaching this ancient healing art to everyone. I now teach about 12 to 15 classes a week, to people of all ages: youngsters and senior citizens, people with arthritis, osteoporosis, back problems, etc.

The physical benefits of yoga are indeed remarkable. People who are young stay younger longer, older people become younger. To see this happening before my very eyes is a joy to behold.

I am no longer using any medication for past physical problems. Arthritis no longer holds fear in me: arteriosclerosis is no longer a threat. My flexibility for a man of my years is, I believe, remarkable. I can glide through a vigorous yoga class. My whole life has changed. I function more and more as I did when I was a much younger person.

One

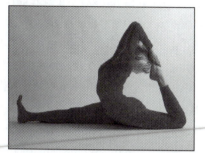

Our Changing View of Aging: How Expectations Determine Outcome

We need to change our idea of what aging is. If I know my biological potential is 130 years, then I don't consider myself middle-aged until I'm 65. . . . One of the great principles of mind/body medicine is that expectancies determine outcome. If you expect to remain strong in old age, you will.

—DEEPAK CHOPRA M.D., *AGELESS BODY, TIMELESS MIND*

As a society and as individuals, we can expect that our notions of aging will continue to change dramatically in the years ahead. Leading pioneers in the field of mind/body medicine such as Deepak Chopra, M.D., an endocrinologist, bestselling author and internationally recognized authority on how our consciousness affects our health, urge us to consider the power that our beliefs about aging have over us. The latest research shows that how we age has more to do with our belief system and mindset about aging than any other factor.

In the last several decades, gerontologists have proved that remaining active throughout life halts the loss of muscle and skeletal tissue. The news is spreading among older people that they should continue all the activities they enjoyed in earlier years—walking, hiking, bicycling, gardening, golf, tennis, karate, swimming, dancing, yoga—you name it. Not long ago, a wild, 100-year-old daredevil named S.L. Potter, defying age, common sense and the fears of his physician and children, made his first bungee jump from a 210-foot tower. Further evidence that we are redefining what is appropriate in old age were photographs in the news of two of America's oldest sisters, Sarah and Elizabeth Delany, then ages 102 and 104—one practicing Shoulderstand, the other stretching in a yoga pose with one foot behind her head.

What happens when we change our old expectations about aging? Gerontologists from Tufts University found out when they put a group of the frailest nursing home residents, ages 87 to 96, on a weight-training regimen. Traditionally doctors believed that this type of elderly person belonged in bed, in a rocker or wheelchair out on the porch or in front of the television. Exercise would exhaust or kill these fragile people. Instead, they thrived. Within eight weeks muscle tone improved by 300 percent. Coordination and balance improved as well. Most important, these elderly people's confidence in being active returned. Some of them who had not been able to walk unassisted could now get up and go to the bathroom

Advanced age is not a static, irreversible biological condition of unwavering decrepitude. Rather, it's a dynamic state that, in most people, can be changed for the better no matter how many years they've lived or neglected their body in the past—Yes, you do have a second chance to right the wrongs you've committed against your body. Your body can be rejuvenated. You can regain vigor, vitality, muscular strength, and aerobic endurance you thought were gone forever . . . this is possible, whether you're middle-aged or pushing 80. The 'markers' of biological aging can be more than altered: in the case of specific physiological functions, they can actually be reversed.

—*William Evans,*
Biomarkers, The 10 Keys
to Prolonging Vitality

by themselves—an act of reclaimed dignity and independence that cannot be underestimated.

With Yoga, the Body Remains Open and Flexible

The accepted view of the aging process has been one of stiffening, rigidity and closing down. Without proper exercise, the body contracts and we lose height, strength and flexibility. As a result, our natural free range of motion is restricted so daily activities become difficult and in some cases impossible. Yoga exercises reverse the aging process by moving each joint in the body through its full range of motion—stretching, strengthening and balancing each part. Most popular forms of weight bearing exercise contract muscles and tighten the musculoskeletal system, adding to the stiffness that normally settles into the body with the passage of time. In our youth-oriented culture, obsessed with thinness, we tighten the muscles to make the body look firmer. What is much more important, however, especially as we grow older, is opening and expanding the body so that the aging process is tempered. Insurance companies, gerontologists, cardiologists, senior exercise physiologists and other health care professionals interested in preventing chronic illness and disability in the older population are becoming increasingly interested in what yoga has to offer older people.

Chronological vs. Biological Age

According to *Age Wave* authors Ken Dychtwald and Joe Flowers, 100 million Americans are changing what

> There is no age limit, one can start yoga when 70 or 80 years old and no damage will occur if the movement comes from the spine. People feel elated and it gives them comfort and encouragement to discover that it is possible for them to control and modify their bodies. To talk about old age as an impediment is an excuse to be lazy.
> —*Vanda Scaravelli, born in 1908, author of* Awakening the Spine

> If we had a culture that nurtured the intelligence implicit in the blood and bone from infancy on, we wouldn't need remedial efforts and there's no telling how far we might advance. Many people have made big changes in later life by learning how to honor the wisdom of their bodies.
> —*Gloria Steinem, who took up weight-training and yoga after age 50, author of* Revolution from Within: A Book of Self-Esteem

How do you define normal? There are people who are biologically 40 and chronologically 80. There are other people who are 20 and their biology reflects the age of 50 or 60. . . . What we call normal aging is the psychopathology of the average. We shouldn't confuse average with normal because there are so many exceptions.

—Deepak Chopra, M.D.,
Ageless Body,
Timeless Mind

we think about aging. Today, there are more older people alive than ever before, and increasing numbers of them are over 85. As the population grows older, we are discovering that chronological age is only one way to measure aging, and perhaps the least accurate one. Chronological age matches what physiologists refer to as our "biological age" only when we are very young. As the years pass by, biological time slows down; the older you are the more slowly you age. By the time we enter midlife, biological age becomes less significant than qualities like zest, energy, enthusiasm, confidence and contentment. In over 20 years of teaching yoga to people of all ages, shapes, sizes and temperaments, I've seen wide variations in the ways human beings change.

In the 1970s, the American Medical Association's Committee on Aging concluded a 10-year study by declaring that it had not found a single physical or mental condition that could be directly attributed to the passage of time. Stress- and diet-related conditions such as high blood pressure, heart disease, arthritis, osteoporosis, loss of muscle strength, reduction in motor fitness (i.e., balance, flexibility, agility, power and reaction time), reduction in respiratory reserves (breathing capacity), constipation and diseases associated with elimination, diabetes, sleep disorders and depression are experienced by young and old alike.

We now know that many of the classic symptoms of aging are caused by inactivity or the wrong type of activity (i.e., mechanical, imbalanced forms of exercise that strain the body), inadequate nutrition and accumulated stress and tension. Even such common outer symptoms of aging—poor posture, rounded shoulders, dowager's hump, closed chest, stiffness and loss of mobility—originate when we are younger and become increasingly pronounced as the years go by.

Health and Aging

Our aging population is increasingly concerned about the availability and affordability of adequate health care. A growing number of people are realizing that what we refer to as our "Health-Care System," which consists primarily of medical doctors, surgeons, drugs and hospitals, should be more accurately labeled as our "Ill-Health-Care System."

Medical services have become very efficient at diagnosing what is wrong with older people. Physician services and the advent of antibiotics have given doctors excellent control of infectious diseases. Hospital and surgical services for illness and injuries have become so proficient that many who would have died at 50, 60 or 70 now live longer.

Many people assume that because the elderly are living longer, they are in good health. Certainly a small percentage of them are, but many aging people suffer from serious and disabling health problems. A closer look at older people who have been saved by modern medicine finds that a high percentage of them are suffering from degenerative diseases. Arthritis, osteoporosis, heart disease, chronic fatigue, cataracts, macular (visual) degeneration, diabetes and cancer are common. While traditional medicine offers drugs, surgery and other methods to treat degenerative diseases, it does not offer the means to prevent them.

Statistics from the U.S. Department of Health and Human Services demonstrate that Americans are not the healthiest people in the world. For example:

Instead of going about the business of healing this sick society, we're lulling it to sleep with services. We need to see services for the aged for what they really are: Novocain. They're not really changing anything. They are simply dulling the pain of loss and deprivation, alienation and frustration and despair, much of what we call senility, and confusion is not organic brain damage but induced by frustration, despair, a sense of loss of purpose and one's role in life.
—Maggie Kuhn, 1970s activist for the elderly

The National Academy of Sciences has reported that if institutionalization could be postponed by just one month, it would save $3 billion in Medicare and Medicaid. And that doesn't include the savings in dignity and independence for elderly people.

—*William Evans,*
Biomarkers, The 10 Keys
to Prolonging Vitality.

- Men in 22 countries have a longer life expectancy
- American women rank seventh in longevity
- Our adult mortality rate is eleventh in the world
- Dental disease affects 98 percent of people of all ages
- Cancer strikes 930,000 Americans annually
- There are 440,000 cancer deaths per year
- Each year 19 million people get heart disease and 750,000 die from it (37 percent of all deaths)
- High blood pressure affects 28 million people
- Arthritis affects 30 million; bursitis affects another 30 million
- Five to 8 million people have asthma, cataracts, diabetes or migraines
- One million people have kidney stones

Eight prescriptions are written each year for every person in the United States, and even more for the elderly. Older people have been known to take as many as 30 different medications during the last year of their life. Each year in the U.S., medication problems are the cause of more than 250,000 hospitalizations for people 65 and older.

People are no longer content to be shuffled from doctor to doctor, only to be told that their illness, pain or degeneration is normal for their age, and to go home, take their medication and get plenty of rest. Our present primary health-care delivery system, which until recently has ignored prevention and health, is failing us at a cost of billions. This is the reason "alternative" health systems are now becoming mainstream. Chiropractic, homeopathy, herbs, acupuncture, massage, nutrition, Ayurvedic medicine, yoga and others are coming into their own as people share positive experiences with these health systems. These more holistic therapies are

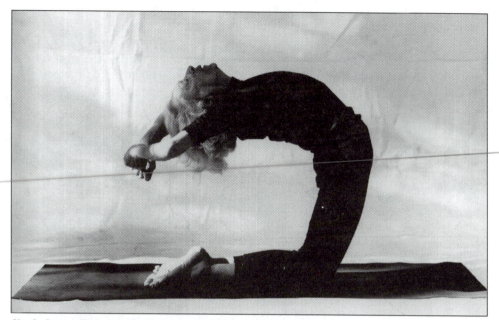

Vanda Scaravelli, in her 80s, is a testament to the benefit of yoga.

safe and generally offer a less expensive means of helping people suffering from many acute and chronic conditions. They are restorative in nature, help to recharge and revitalize the body's precious stores of energy, and thus help to prevent illness, disease and degeneration.

Yoga offers a uniquely holistic approach to health. This ancient science, with its deep roots in Ayurvedic medicine, is truly the most complete system of self-health care that exists. The best part of it is that it is something you do to yourself, for yourself. It is an active, rather than a passive, approach to keeping yourself healthy and fit.

As I grow older, it is liberating and exhilarating to feel more freedom of movement, openness and extension in my joints and muscles than back in my younger years. As a teacher, I find it a continual revelation to see how the bodies of people of all ages respond to yoga and proper exercise.

Ayurveda, "the science of life" or "knowledge of life span" in Sanskrit, is a 5,000 year-old system of mind/body medicine.

Betty Eiler: After 50, Include Yoga in Your Lifestyle

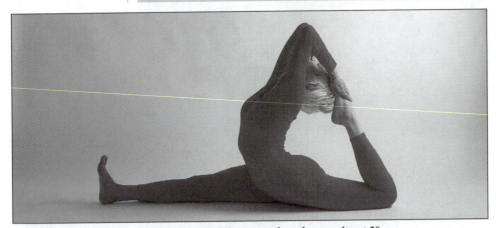

Betty Eiler is a yoga teacher who began practicing yoga when she was almost 50.

My general health, well-being and joy in life have increased immeasurably. It seems to me that the most important thing that seniors can do to enhance their lives is to change their lifestyle to include yoga with experienced and qualified instructors. To have it work for each of us, we must DO IT frequently.

I have had many inspiring experiences working with students over the age of 50. They involve all aspects of healing, including reduction of rheumatoid arthritis; recovery from frequent headaches, numbness in hands; backaches; and remission of multiple sclerosis.

Those who have the discipline to stay for six months or more report their increased feeling of well-being and enthusiasm for life. Their range of movement increases dramatically, enabling many to return to physical activities they thought were lost forever: gardening, climbing uphill, biking, reaching and bending, and simply sitting comfortably on the floor.

The wonderful progress people in this age range make has inspired me to start taking "before" pictures of the ones I believe will make a commitment to yoga. After six months or so, we can document their progress with "after" pictures. The changes might be dramatic or subtle. People often forget how they felt or looked pre-yoga.

As for myself, I began yoga approximately 13 years ago, and some of the changes I have experienced are:

- My mild scoliosis disappeared.
- My shoe size slowly moved from a 6½ N to now an 8½ N or B, and the flat footprints of my childhood are now footprints with arches.
- My seated poses, such as sitting with the soles of my feet together *(Baddha Konasana)*, were once with rounded back and knees very elevated. My knees now touch the floor without wall support (on a stretched-out day).
- I am comfortable doing the Lotus in Headstand *(Pindasana)*.
- At age 52, for the first time in my life, I did the Splits *(Hanumasana)*, and at age 55 I did a mid-room, Full Arm Balance *(Adho Mukha Vrksasana)*, dropping back to the Upward Bow *(Urdhva Dhanurasana)*.

For people over 50 thinking about starting yoga I say, "Try it, you'll like it." Live life with excitement and enthusiasm and do something different. You will be amazed how the body responds. I find a new awareness in every class I attend —a subtle opening that I didn't have the last time I did a certain posture, a reaching for the ceiling and feeling that I'm getting there. I have become more centered and have a greater amount of stamina and physical strength. This, too, is because of the guidance of the Inner Spirit.

—Marleen Burrow, a student of Betty Eiler

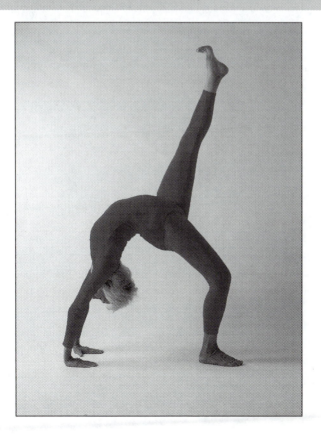

Two

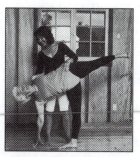

How Yoga Slows Down and Reverses the Aging Process

Yoga deals with the most profound of mysteries, the essential nature of the human being in relation to the universe. The meaning of Yoga is union or yoking, from the Sanskrit "yug," to unite. In the context of yoga philosophy, the union is between the individual soul and universal soul. The individual has to search for the divine within, and Yoga provides the systematic steps to achieve this.

—SILVA MEHTA, *YOGA: THE IYENGAR WAY*

Yoga: The Ideal Health System for People Over 50

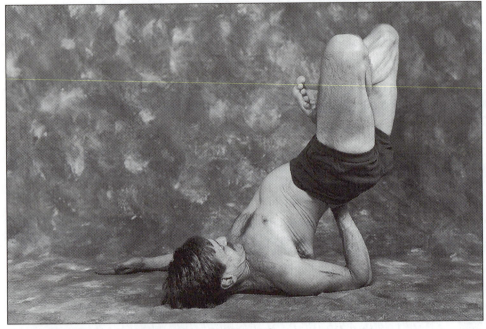

Jim Jacobs, in his 50s, practices Lotus Pose in Shoulderstand.

It's interesting to me how yoga is becoming incredibly popular. . . . We are really living in a very complex time—a time of great turmoil and change. The more irrational of us are worried about the millennium ending—as if a date would really matter. Yoga is a good antidote for all that. Yoga will take us out of all this historical paranoia. It's a long haul we're in.

—Sting (Interview with Ganga White, Yoga Journal, November/December 1995)

Yoga philosophy has appealed to great thinkers for centuries and today, as we head into the 21st century, it is evident that yoga is becoming more and more a part of our lifestyle. Millions of Americans from all walks of life practice yoga, and the popularity of this ageless, timeless, holistic health system will flourish even more as modern medicine rediscovers and documents its value.

Dean Ornish, M.D., author of *Dr. Dean Ornish's Program for Reversing Heart Disease*, and other renowned medical specialists recommend yoga as a key part of a program for preventing and reversing heart disease. Most of today's stress management techniques have their roots in yoga. Hospitals throughout the country are using yoga and meditation to help patients suffering from chronic pain and stress-related medical disorders. Doctors at Cedars-Sinai Medical Center in Los Angeles are so certain of yoga's health benefits that it is a key part of their program for people who have had heart attacks. C. Noel Bairey Merz, a cardiologist there, states emphatically, "The bottom line is that yoga is an exercise that is good for the heart."

If you are new to yoga, let me assure you that whatever your age or physical condition and whatever your religious belief or cultural heritage, the practice of yoga's stretching and strengthening exercises and the breathing and relaxation techniques can help you to vastly improve the quality of your life and health.

The word "healing" comes from the root, "to make whole." The word "yoga" comes from the Sanskrit, meaning to yoke or discipline, to unite, to make whole. Because true health involves body, mind and spirit, yoga incorporates physiological, psychological and spiritual processes. There are various systems of yoga, and each provides different ways of unifying the physical, mental, emotional and spiritual aspects of a human being.

Yoga is not a religion. It is a nonsectarian method for promoting a healthy and harmonious lifestyle. Any person of any faith can practice yoga and find his or her religion enhanced as a result.

What Is Hatha Yoga?

This book focuses on hatha yoga—a physical discipline that explores the intimate connection between the body, mind and spirit. The Sanskrit word *ha* means "sun" and *tha* means "moon." The goal of hatha yoga is

When I go into gyms and health clubs, I see men with rounded shoulders use a weight machine and do 50 lifts that tend to round the shoulders and three lifts that tend to open the chest. The lifts that open the chest are hard for them to do and, hence, are not as pleasing psychologically; so they don't do many. But what they don't know is that the pleasing lifts are reinforcing all the negative patterns about their bodies: rounding their shoulders, collapsing their lungs, curtailing their breathing. What they need is somebody to show them how to open their bodies to oxygen, work with alignment, and exercise for health.
—Sue Luby, fitness expert, yoga teacher and author of Bodysense: The Hazard-Free Fitness Program for Men and Women

to balance and unify the positive and negative energy flows (life forces) within the body. Using the flow of the breath and the internal flow of these energies, yoga helps us to realize our potential for health and self-healing.

All of the approaches to hatha yoga involve the practice of various movements and postures. In general, they consist of forward bends, backbends, twists, inversions, standing and balancing poses as well as relaxation and breathing techniques. These movements and postures, along with conscious use of the breath, remove stiffness and tension from the body, restore vitality, strength and stamina, and improve balance and coordination; they also promote the efficiency of the body processes of digestion, assimilation and detoxification.

Older people, in particular, need a conscious, intelligent, expansive and non-mechanical approach to exercise that involves the whole person—body, mind and spirit. At the physical level, the practice of yoga strengthens and balances all the systems of the body; yoga also offers relief from the various ailments mistakenly attributed to aging. From the mental or psychological viewpoint, yoga improves concentration, calms and steadies the emotions and helps the practitioner to see life with greater perspective. In the realm of the spiritual, yoga expands awareness and teaches the mind and body to be quiet and at peace. Yoga has a unique place in our search for health because it offers a practical technique for experiencing unity and harmony of every aspect of our being.

According to yogic tradition, the years after 50 are the ideal time for psychological and spiritual growth. The practice of yoga not only restores the health and vitality of the body, but the philosophy behind yoga aims to open and expand a human being on all levels so that aging can become a time of greater perspective and illumination, rather than deterioration.

Yoga Prevents and Corrects the Most Visible Symptom of Aging— the Rounding of the Spine

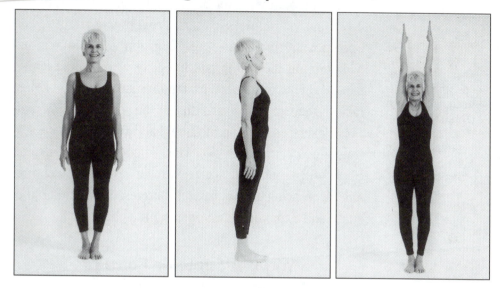

Yoga prevents and can even reverse the most visible and obvious symptom of aging—one that cannot be disguised or transformed cosmetically—the shortening and rounding of the spine. In our culture, where people spend years hunched over a desk or steering wheel, or engaged in other activities that tend to pull our upper body forward, a rounded upper back, forward head and collapsed chest are so prevalent among people over the age of 50 that we almost consider it a normal part of aging.

Over the course of a "normal" lifetime, the spine degenerates and the body becomes shorter. When the back becomes rounded, it compresses the chest, which causes shallow breathing. By limiting the amount of oxygen the cells receive, this 'old age posture' contributes to cardiovascular and other health problems. Yoga counteracts and reverses all of this.

Poor posture and the degeneration of the spinal column affect the health of every system of the body. Not only do a rounded back and collapsed chest restrict breathing, but they interfere with the vital flow of blood and of nerve impulses to the internal organs. In this way poor posture interferes with digestion and elimination. Maintaining the health and integrity of the spine is the central theme of yoga. With regular practice, yoga helps restore the strength and agility of the spine, slowing and even reversing the common degenerative changes often found in people over 50. The practice guides in this book will teach you specific exercises for preventing and decreasing upper back roundness, elongating the spine and expanding and opening the chest.

Yoga: A Superior Form of Weight-Bearing Exercise for Preventing Osteoporosis

In the last 20 years, scientists have learned how important exercise is to maintaining the strength of the bones. During weight-bearing exercise, muscles transmit mechanical and bioelectrical signals to the bone, causing it to thicken. Research has found that daily weight-bearing exercise is crucial to helping both women and men avoid osteoporosis, or porous, brittle bones. In a person with severe osteoporosis, a fall, blow or lifting action that would not affect the average person can easily cause one or more bones to break.

Medical textbooks and articles about exercise frequently claim that yoga is not a weight-bearing exercise and is therefore not considered effective for strengthening bones and preventing osteoporosis. Yoga's stretching exercises are wrongfully relegated to the role of warming up the body for other physical activities or helping to cool it down afterwards.

In fact, yoga is a superior form of weight-bearing exercise because it stimulates bones throughout the

Posture affects every system of the body—not only the neuro-muscular system (joints, ligaments, bones, muscles and the nerves that move them), but the endocrine system (pituitary, thyroid, adrenal, etc.) and the cardiovascular, circulatory and respiratory system. All of these systems can be directly correlated and related to problems with posture.

—Nikolaas Tinbergen, 1973 Nobel laureate in Physiology/Medicine

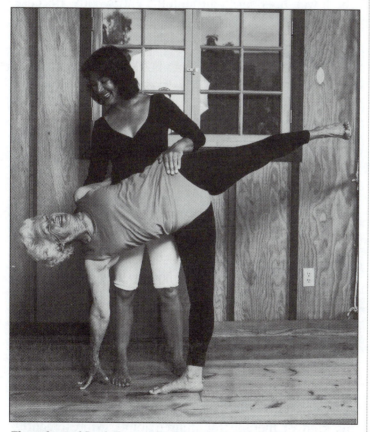

The author and Sandy Yost, age 72, demonstrating the Half-Moon Pose. This standing position stimulates the bones of the legs, arms and spine to retain calcium. Beginners can practice this pose with their hand on a block or chair, their back against a wall or counter, or with the help of a teacher or friend, as illustrated.

body. In yoga's flowing, graceful movements, weight is systematically applied to bones in the hands, arms, upper body, neck and even the head, as well as the feet and legs. Inverted weight-bearing yoga postures such as Handstands and Headstands, where the bones in the arms, wrists and hands are strengthened by supporting the weight of one's own body, all work to prevent osteoporosis and other problems related to a weak skeletal structure. Yoga is one of the few exercise systems in which weight is borne through the entire body. Because yoga postures are learned gradually, the weight applied to the bones increases safely, incrementally, as the student becomes stronger and can hold postures for longer periods of time. This is especially important after the age of 50. (See chapter 7 on osteoporosis.)

Keeping Your Joints Young

While yoga is already known for restoring our natural, youthful flexibility, most people are not aware of yoga's therapeutic effect on the joints. When a joint is injured, one of the first rehabilitation techniques in physical therapy is called passive range of motion. In passive range of motion, the therapist moves the joint as far as possible without pain. Through many repetitions of the movement, the range of motion is gradually increased. The patient then graduates to active range of motion exercise, doing the same maneuvers without assistance.

Western medicine has long recognized the value of this kind of therapy for injured joints. More recently, however, physicians are realizing that the same principle, which is the basis of much of the work done in yoga, helps prevent the degeneration of healthy joints.

Health is reflected in lifestyle, and if we ignore our bodies we may, even by our mid-thirties, stiffen far more than necessary. Movement lubricates the muscles, ligaments, and joints. If we become sedentary, the muscles lose tone and the muscle groups that hold us upright become unevenly matched. The joints then feel strain, lose space in which to articulate, and we start to suffer from wear and tear. At this point we become less inclined to move because it is not comfortable to do so. This is premature aging. Stretching daily can reduce this stiffness, allowing us eventually to dance, play tennis, and enjoy our bodies well into our real old age.

—*Maxine Tobias,*
Complete Stretching

Inverted Poses: The Fountain of Youth

Newcomers to yoga are usually fascinated—and sometimes put off—by the sight of their more experienced classmates hanging upside down from wall ropes like bats or going upside down in Handstand, Headstand or another inverted position. Naturally, they want to know about the benefits of inverting the body.

Physicians have long recognized the beneficial effects of reversing the downward pull of gravity on the circulation, lungs and brain. They frequently advise their patients to put their feet up to compensate for the weakening of veins in the lower legs of many older people. Doctors have also reversed gravity in the treatment of respiratory problems. For example, a method called "posture drainage" predates antibiotics for treating certain lung infections. Using this technique, the patient assumes various positions to turn various parts of the lungs (which are arranged like the branches of a tree) upside down. However, the most effective form of postural drainage is one not yet commonly described by Western medicine: that of turning the body upside down, as in the inverted yoga postures.

The gravitational force of the earth is among the most powerful physical influences on the human body. Just as plants and trees are shaped by the direction of sunlight and wind, our bodies are shaped by the pull of gravity. As time goes by, the body has a tendency to narrow at the top and settle toward the bottom. Reversing the downward pull of gravity helps the body retain its balance and symmetry.

Gravity also tends to cause the compression and flattening of the cells and blood vessels of the brain, and the collapse of the top lobes of the lungs. It also tends to create stress and strain on the ligaments, blood vessels and organs in the abdominal cavity. Being upside down helps to reverse all these tendencies. The large intestines are especially responsive to the relief from gravitational compression, and inverted poses are an effective treatment for constipation.

To further appreciate the benefits of reversing gravity, consider the obvious fact that water always flows downhill. The fluids that comprise 75 to 80 percent of our body are generally at the mercy of gravity, and the circulatory system must constantly adjust to gravity's effects. One of the most vital functions of the cardiovascular system is to deliver fresh blood to the brain. When we are in a horizontal position, the heart is at the same level as the brain, and gravity has little effect on the flow of blood between the brain and the heart. When we are standing or sitting, the brain is above the heart and the cardiovascular system must compensate by working harder to pump blood to the brain. In a partially or fully inverted position, the brain is below the level of the heart and gravity pulls blood into the brain; the brain receives a proper blood supply with minimum effort by the heart.

When the body is completely inverted, venous blood flows from the legs and abdomen to the heart without strain. According to yoga experts and doctors studying yoga, the regular and long-term practice of forward bends and inversions can reduce arterial blood pressure by helping to reset the pressure regulating reflexes. The Headstand helps to increase venous return to the heart, bringing the deoxygenated blood toward the heart and relieving pressure in the passive venous system caused by the pooling of blood in the legs during standing.

During the course of a typical day, most people spend 16 or more hours with the head (brain) above the heart and the legs and pelvic area below the heart. I always advise students who are not yet ready to practice more difficult upside-down positions to at least put their legs up against a wall for five minutes. Inverted positions, especially when combined with proper nutritional support, can alleviate problems with varicose veins and, if begun in time, can prevent them.

Reversing Gravity Reverses the Aging Process

It is well known among yoga practitioners that the inverted yoga positions slow down and even reverse the common physical changes that come with the passage of time.

Turning the body even halfway upside down by bending forward from a standing position increases the circulation to the entire upper body, including the brain. The revitalizing and relaxing effect of standing forward bends and completely inverted positions is related, in part, to this change. When the body is inverted, blood circulates easily around the neck, chest and head. This increased circulation stimulates the thyroid and parathyroid glands and helps the lungs, throat and sinuses become resistant to infection. It is also possible that inversions have a positive effect on the brain, as we come out of these postures feeling invigorated and clear-headed.

My early interest in yoga was kindled by a 60-year-old-teacher who told me that she discovered yoga about the time she put her mother and mother-in-law in a rest home. She explained, "The agony of taking them to a

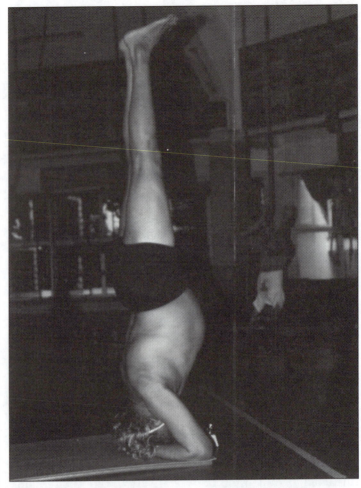

B.K.S. Iyengar at age 75. Inverted poses revitalize the whole body.

rest home after they were senile made a profound impression on me. I began to consider that perhaps I could hold back or maybe even prevent senility by increasing the flow of blood to my brain through the inverted postures."

The ravages of senility are apparent in every nursing home in the country. While Western medicine accepts the fact that this is a degenerative disease associated with inadequate circulation to the brain, researchers have found few effective ways of preventing or treating it. The blood flow to the brain gradually reduces as one grows older. Dr. Krishna Raman, in his writings on yoga and the circulatory system, states that by the time a person is 65, the blood flow to the brain may be a third of what it was at age 25. Yoga teaches that the most effective way of increasing blood to the brain is to allow gravity to do the work for you by bringing the brain below the level of the heart, permitting circulation to the upper body to increase without putting strain on the heart.

After age 50, it becomes increasingly important to reverse the downward pull of gravity on the body.

Precautions on Practicing Inversions

Inverted positions, whether done with special equipment, pelvic swings, antigravity devices or your own upper body strength, are only as safe as people are educated to make them. Inverted positions like the Headstand should be learned under the guidance of an experienced teacher and should not be practiced by individuals with the following conditions: high blood pressure; glaucoma; detached retina; heart problems or stroke; epilepsy, seizures, or other brain disorders; acute infections of the ear, throat or sinuses; osteoporosis; obesity; conditions requiring aspirin therapy; chronic neck problems or whiplash. These conditions may improve with gentle supported forward bends and supported inversions.

Chapter 11 describes simple Legs-Up-the-Wall Pose and other inverted positions that most people new to yoga can safely practice.

Joyce Rudduck: No One Is Ever Too Old or Too Stiff to Do Yoga

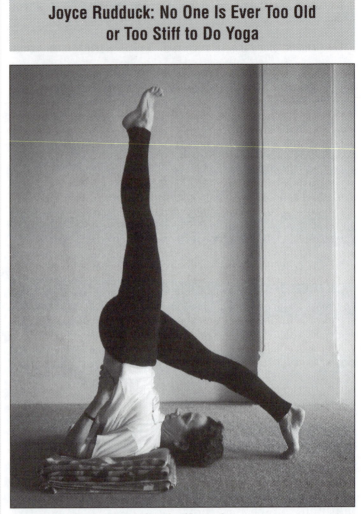

Joyce Rudduck in the rejuvenating Shoulderstand.

Joyce Rudduck, who is in her 60s, is co-director and teacher at the Australian School of Yoga. She began practicing yoga at 54 as a last resort to ease the constant pain she still suffered from two accidents years ago. In one accident, a crowbar fell on her head, injuring her neck. A year later she was thrown from a turning truck and jammed her lower back.

The doctor told me, "You will just have to learn to live with it," but my interior self said, "No, I will not!" I had always been a very active person, but the growing pain throughout my body was gradually slowing me down. In every position, I was always shifting to get out of pain. Because of the accidents, I was always suffering and in pain.

At last I had the good fortune to be referred to an excellent physical therapist who asked, "Joyce, have you ever done yoga?" I explained that I'd gone to a few classes a few years ago and that it felt fine but nothing to rave about. However, she persisted, saying that this was a different approach to yoga. She described it as "therapeutic yoga," and told me to think about it.

After mulling it over for a week I decided to give it a whirl, telling myself that I had nothing to lose. At that point I was desperate and willing to try anything.

Thus I arrived at the Australian School of Yoga. I remember well the first things we did in that class. We lay on our back, feet to the wall, and stretched our legs this way and that with straps. Our instructor was the late Martyn Jackson, one of B.K.S. Iyengar's advanced senior teachers. His big cheery voice boomed out over everyone. Every moment was agony! Our shoulders were opened by lying on our stomachs with our hands raised up on chairs. His instructions were "five minutes before breakfast—five minutes before your supper every day."

Obediently I complied and months later reaped the reward. That was in November 1985.

After the first six months I began coming to class twice a week. After a year, four times a week—and so I grew into yoga.

Then I developed an ardent desire to ease the pain of others. No one in my opinion was too old, too stiff or too anything to do yoga because I had done it and was still doing it and improving all the time.

In 1986 Martyn began a weekday 6 A.M. intensive class, which I attended every day before work. It was hard, but rewarding. Fear was dissolving, my whole being was changing physically and mentally. Slowly I began to feel a new me. The constant pain was disappearing.

In 1988 I took a teacher's training course. For a "stiffy over 50," it is not an easy road, but with determination and perseverance and doing something quietly every day no matter how small, one grows and blossoms and learns that, "Your body is the teacher," and teachers become guiding lights to assist you.

Three

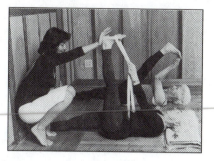

In Praise of Props

How Common Household Objects Can Help You Improve Your Posture, Maintain Your Balance, and Stretch, Strengthen and Relax

Props are silent instructors that teach directly to the intelligence of the body, and through that direct perception the harmony of mind, body and spirit can be experienced.

—Mary Dunn, YOGA TEACHER

Most of us think we don't have enough time to exercise. What a distorted paradigm! We don't have time not to. We're talking about three to six hours a week or a minimum of 30 minutes a day, every other day. That hardly seems like an inordinate amount of time considering the tremendous benefits in terms of the impact on the other 162-165 hours of the week.

—STEPHEN R. COVEY, *THE 7 HABITS OF HIGHLY EFFECTIVE PEOPLE*

Back in the 1960s, when Westerners first began turning to yoga, the use of a prop to practice yoga was practically unheard of. Potential yogis simply came to class with an exercise mat, a blanket or beach towel. Everyone mimicked the teacher's demonstration of the yoga positions as best he or she could. You were not expected to sweat or be perfect. As I recall, emphasis was on deep relaxation in the corpse pose. Classes were often held by candlelight, with incense and Indian sitar music to evoke a mystical atmosphere.

Nowadays, at the turn of the 21st century, when you walk into a yoga classroom, you will likely see folding chairs and benches stacked in one corner of the room and shelves filled with blankets, nonskid mats, pillows and bolsters of various shapes and sizes, wooden blocks, dowels and 10-pound sandbags. There may also be ropes, straps, pelvic slings or other anti-gravity equipment hanging from the walls or suspended from the ceiling. You may see a whale-shaped piece of furniture—a unique wooden object known as a backbending bench.

If you arrive early, some students will probably be sitting or lying down quietly, but others are using these props, also known as yoga tools or yoga aids, to warm

This is the single most powerful investment we can ever make in life—investment in ourselves, in the only instrument we have with which to deal with life and to contribute.

—*Stephen R. Covey, The 7 Habits of Highly Effective People*

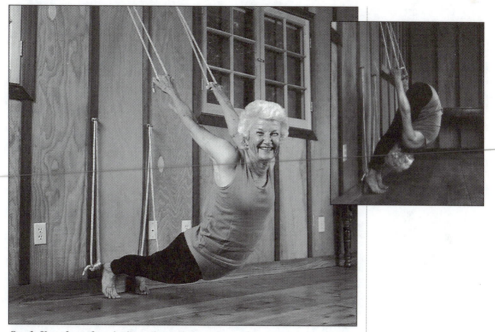

Sandy Yost shows how invigorating using ropes can be.

up or to relax before class starts. People of all ages are hanging halfway or completely upside down from ropes, and those that aren't reversing gravity are lying on the floor, stretching their legs with a strap around one foot. Other students are lying over bolsters, benches and chairs. Some are sitting on top of a block or bolsters with the soles of their feet together and sandbags weighing down their thighs.

According to Ruth Steiger and Kay Eskenazi, co-founders of the company Yoga Props and authors of the *Yoga Prop Usage Guides* (see Resources), "A prop is any object that helps you to stretch, strengthen, relax or improve your body alignment. By providing more height, weight or support, props help you to extend beyond habitual limitations and teach you that your body is capable of doing much more than you think it can!"

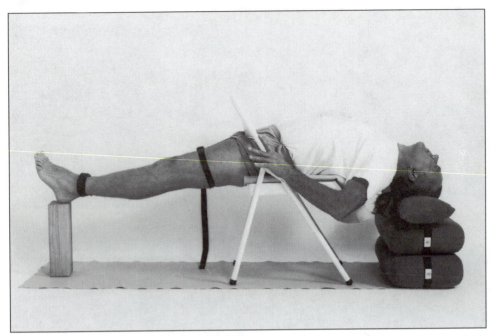

Props are adapted to a student's body type and flexibility.

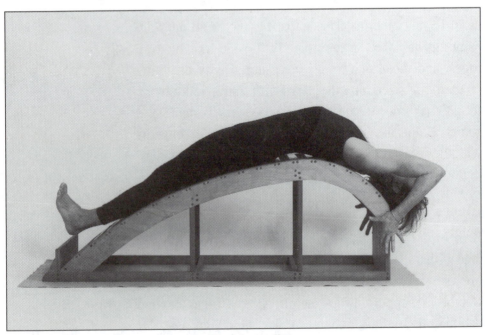

The backbending bench allows you to stretch with minimum effort.

Using yoga props makes postures safer and more accessible. Since many people are already stiff by the time they start yoga, props allow them to practice poses they would not ordinarily be able to do.

People over 50 also frequently come to yoga with problems, ranging from back and neck pain or knee problems to old injuries. The more problems a student has, the more useful yoga props are. Props allow you to hold poses longer, so you can experience their healing effects. By supporting the body in the yoga posture, muscles can lengthen in a passive, non-strenuous way. The use of props also helps to improve blood circulation and breathing capacity.

For example, if you cannot bend forward and bring your hands to the floor without straining or bending your knees, try placing your hands on a desk, table or chair. As you become more flexible you will find that you can put your hands on a lower prop like a bench, a stack of books or a block. With practice, most people's hands will touch the floor and the prop will no longer be necessary.

The creative use of props expands the help a teacher can give, especially when teaching classes of various levels of ability. In a group situation, for example, those students who are not strong enough to practice inversions on their own can safely receive their benefits by being supported by ropes suspended from the wall or ceiling. The ropes absorb some or all of a student's weight, inversions can be performed without strain, and the student can receive the benefits of the pose.

Props are also used to teach students how a pose done correctly should feel. A rope hanging from a wall hook or doorknob and placed at the top of the legs in *Adho Mukha Svanasana,* the Downward-Facing Dog Pose, allows the student to stretch the torso and arms as far forward as possible. Because the rope pulls the student's weight back into the legs, it helps the student experience the elongation of the abdomen and the deep muscles of the torso in the pose. The head can rest on a bolster or pillow. In this way, a wonderful, passive stretch is experienced. The student gets a taste of what it feels like to "let go" in a pose, to relax and enjoy the pose. Use of the props facilitates imprinting of the correct action in the pose so that the student understands it when the prop has been removed.

By using props, students who need to conserve their energy can practice more strenuous poses without overexerting themselves. People with chronic illness can use props to practice without undue strain and fatigue.

Props are adapted to a student's body type and flexibility. They are especially helpful to anyone who may avoid trying certain poses because of fear, problems with balance such as loss of hearing and eyesight, pain and various other limitations. In therapeutic situations, props are invaluable. People who have scoliosis (curvature of the spine), rounded back or other chronic postural problems can significantly improve their posture by stretching with the help of a prop.

Props give tremendous encouragement, create confidence, reduce pain, support the body and guide students to practice the poses correctly. In addition to using common objects around the house as props, a wide range of professionally designed yoga props are available and well worth the cost.

Sitting Comfortably on the Floor

A lifetime of sitting in chairs causes stiffness in the hips and knees. As such, most people unaccustomed to

sitting on the floor tend to slump backwards and collapse their chest. By sitting on two firmly folded blankets, a bolster, a big book or other height, older adults
can quickly learn what it feels like to sit on the floor
with their back straight and chest open.

The stiffer you are in the hips, the thicker the height
under your bottom should be. If you feel strain in your
knees, try placing a folded blanket or other support
under your knees.

How Chairs Support Your Yoga Practice

The prop I use most frequently in classes for beginners over 50 is an ordinary, metal folding chair. The best
folding chair to use is very stable and sturdy, with a
level seat that does not collapse when you put weight on
it, and it has a wide space in between the backrest and
the seat. If you can find one with a rung between the
back legs, that would be helpful, but if this type is not
readily available, just find a chair that matches the first
part of this description as closely as possible.

While other armless chairs can also be used for yoga,
standard metal folding chairs are more versatile. They
may be used for supported restorative postures and backbends. If you don't have access to a folding chair at the
moment, use the plainest, sturdiest armless chair in your
house. Avoid cushioned or upholstered chairs, since they
do not provide a firm, even base of support. An inexpen-
sive folding chair can be used in a multitude of ways to
stretch and strengthen your body in ways that challenge
the most sophisticated gym equipment. You can bend
forward, backward and sideways, do push-ups, relieve

backaches and shoulder aches, and go upside down safely with the assistance of this simple piece of furniture.

Chairs can be used in dozens of innovative ways. They allow new students to practice poses that are often too challenging for beginners of any age—but chairs are especially useful for students over 50. Many of my older students initially practice yoga standing poses with the help of a chair or wall. Safety is another important reason for using walls or chairs, especially for beginners over 60 or 70. These props help older people with balance problems practice yoga without slipping or falling. In this way, props help build confidence and stamina. The energy that you might normally divert into struggling to keep your balance can be channeled into practicing the poses correctly and holding them longer. As the poses become more familiar, most students develop the balance to practice without a wall or chair.

Yoga Sitting on a Chair

In cases where sitting or lying on the floor is really not possible or practical, the use of one or two chairs to sit on can be helpful. A folded sticky mat prevents the student from being uncomfortable or, in cases where muscles are very weak, from sliding out of the chair. The surface of the chair becomes a floor, without the hassle of getting up and down off the floor, for someone who does not have sufficient strength in the stomach and back muscles to keep the body erect. A blanket on top of the sticky mat allows the person to sit forward on the sitting bones, keeping the spine in an elongated position.

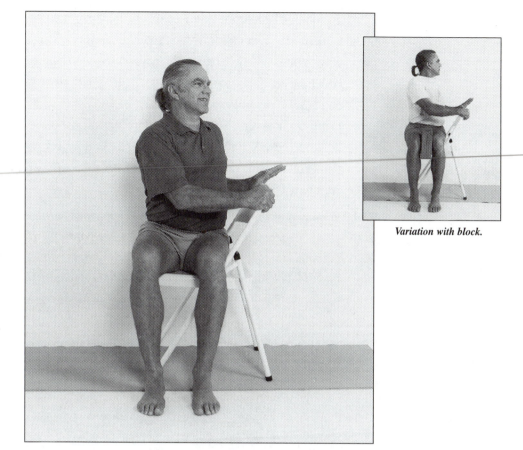

Variation with block.

Jay Myers, a new student in his 50s, feels the benefit of this simple Chair Twist.

Chair Twist

1. Sit sideways on the whole seat of a chair, with the right hip against the back of the chair.
2. Pressing your feet firmly into the floor, lift your rib cage, stretch your shoulders back and down, and lengthen your spine upward. Keep your knees straight in line with your feet.
3. Continue pressing your feet firmly into the floor as you turn to hold the back of the chair. Pull with the left hand to bring the left side of the body toward

the back of the chair, and push with the right hand to turn the right side away from the chair. Keep your upper body stretching toward the ceiling as you turn to the maximum. Turn your head slowly and look over your right shoulder.

4. Continue twisting for several more breaths; exhale as you come back to the center. Pause for a moment, sitting tall. Move to the opposite side of the chair to repeat on your left side.

Note: If your feet do not reach the floor when seated in the chair, place a block, stool or other height under your feet. If your feet and knees tend to splay out when twisting, hold a block or book between your knees as illustrated on page 35.

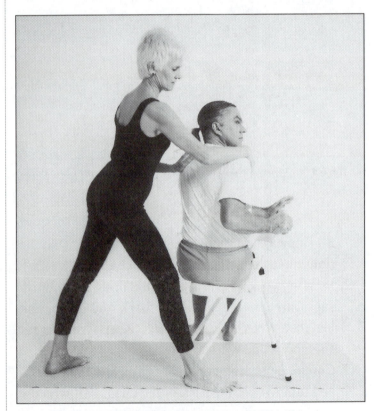

Yoga teacher Betty Eiler helps her student turn more in Chair Twist.

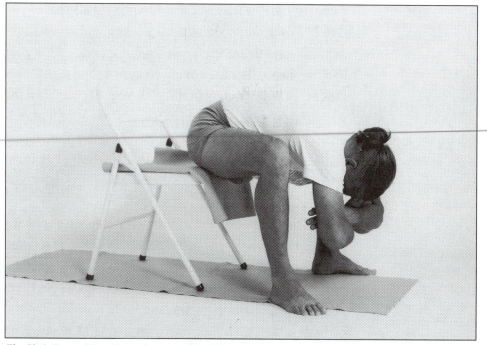

The Chair Forward Bend is a refreshing pick-me-up.

Chair Forward Bend

After the Chair Twist, it is very restful to sit on the front of the chair. Spread the legs wide apart, press firmly into the floor with your feet and stretch your trunk upward. Slowly bend forward, relaxing the back and the head. You can hold your elbows as illustrated, or place your hands on a stool, bolster or the floor.

The Wall: Your Best At-Home Teacher

One of the best yet most overlooked props for stretching is the wall. "The wall is your best guru—it doesn't lie!" my teachers told me when I first began yoga. I recommend that you start your at-home practice by making sure you have at least six feet of empty wall space. Use it to help you understand good posture and body alignment by practicing the yoga standing poses with your back against it. For improving posture, spend a few minutes every day standing "tall" with your back against the wall. If you tend to stoop forward, stretch your shoulders back and down the wall several times a day. You can also use a counter, railing or sturdy table, as illustrated on page 39, to remind you how healthy, open posture feels.

Students who come to class with balance problems can gain strength and confidence by first practicing Triangle Pose and other vital weight-bearing standing poses with their back against a wall. In cases where it has become difficult to maintain an upright position, the use of both a wall and wall ropes (available at many yoga centers or from a yoga prop source) are invaluable for rebuilding strength and stamina. Standing poses can also be practiced by bracing the back foot against a wall and holding wall ropes, as illustrated on page 39. I especially encourage my older beginners who find it difficult to maintain their balance in the middle of the room to practice standing poses at home with the support of a wall, sturdy table, railing or kitchen counter.

How to Practice Triangle Pose at a Wall (Trikonasana)

1. Stand tall with your posture open, shoulders relaxed away from your ears, near a wall. Step your feet about three-and-a-half to four feet apart (depending on the length of your legs), keeping your feet in line, facing forward, heels close to the wall.

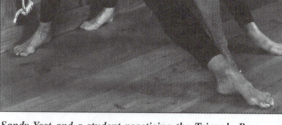

Sandy Yost and a student practicing the Triangle Pose with wall ropes. Walls and wall ropes help students gain strength and confidence.

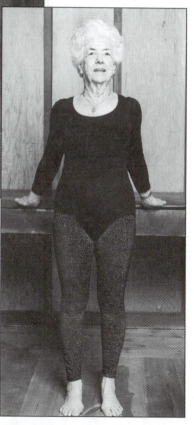

This simple stance immediately gives you a more youthful posture.

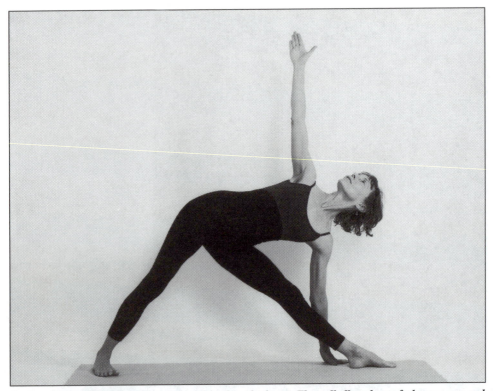

Barbara Wiechmann, in her 50s, is grateful for the gift of yoga. The wall allows her to feel more open and relaxed in the Triangle Pose.

2. Breathe normally. Anchor and root your feet to the earth by pressing the soles of your feet deep into the floor. Activate your legs by pulling up the thigh muscles. Allow your body to become taller and taller, lengthening your spine upward. Raise your arms to shoulder level, palms facing down, and stretch out through your fingertips. Feel the center of your body expand and open.

3. When you feel stable and centered in this position, turn the left foot about 15 degrees in, and the right foot 90 degrees out. Line up the right heel directly in line with the center of the left arch.

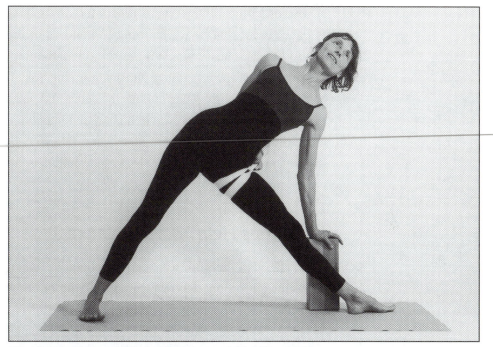

Triangle Pose. The use of a block and strap opens the shoulders and hips.

4. Inhale, and on exhalation stretch to the right from the hip joint, so your torso bends sideways as a unit toward your right leg. In the beginning you may need to place your right hand on your leg, a chair or block. Extend your left arm up, in line with the right arm, palm facing forward. If you feel unusual strain in your shoulder, try placing your left hand on your hip.

5. Stay in the pose for several breaths, keeping your legs active, shoulders and neck relaxed. Come out of the pose on an inhalation, keeping your body close to the wall. Turn your feet to face forward. Relax back into the wall and pause for a moment to feel the effects of the pose. Repeat on the other side.

The use of a block and strap, as illustrated on the previous page, is invaluable for learning to bend from the hip joint with the chest open and the spine lengthening.

Standing poses are refreshing and invigorating for all ages and levels of ability. They remove the aches and pains of "old age." They also improve circulation and breathing, stimulate digestion, regulate the kidneys and relieve constipation. The back, hips, knees, neck and shoulders all gain strength and mobility with regular practice.

Props Help You to Balance

Walls are also helpful for learning balance when standing upright on one leg or turning halfway or completely upside down, as described in chapters 4 and 11.

My older students report that practicing balance poses such as the Tree Pose in class helps them improve their balance in daily life. To build strength and confidence, Tree Pose can first be practiced standing near a wall for support. The wall reminds students to maintain good posture while balancing in the pose. Beginners tend to hunch their shoulders forward when attempting to place their foot against their inner thigh. Practicing with a strap around the ankle of the lifted leg, as illustrated on the next page, is useful for keeping the foot from slipping and for maintaining healthy, open posture in the pose. In addition to giving a sense of balance, Tree Pose strengthens the feet and legs.

Tree Pose

1. The ability to balance on one foot starts by learning to stand firm on both feet, rooted to the earth.

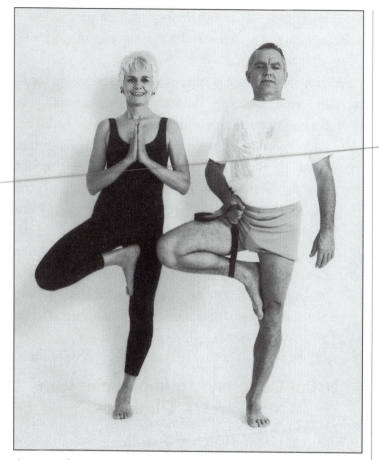

A strap can keep your foot from slipping in this balance pose.

Stand tall with your feet and knees facing forward.
Be aware that the feet are your foundation when
you stand. Create stability while you have both feet
on the ground. Feel the contact of the soles of your
feet on the floor. As awareness of your body deepens, the soles of the feet feel increasingly sensitive
and alive, like the palms of your hands on the floor.

2. Standing firm on the left leg, bend the right leg to
the side. Catch the ankle (or wrap a strap around
your ankle) and place the foot at the top of the left

inner thigh. Bring your foot as high up the leg as possible. Press the right knee back, in line with your hip.

3. Tree Pose can be practiced with the arms and hands in various positions. Whether you practice with your hands in prayer position as illustrated, or with your arms stretching upward above your head, allow your chest to lift and open, your spine to lengthen upward. Stay steady by continuously firming and anchoring the standing leg. Soften your eyes, focus your gaze. Find your balance. To release out of the pose, bring the arms and leg down. Pause for a moment, standing steady on both feet. Repeat on the other side. *Note: If you feel unusual strain bringing the sole of your foot against your inner thigh, try practicing with your foot lower down the leg.*

Using Doorways to Improve Posture and Stretch Shoulders

I never tire of showing my students the many uses of a doorway and the door frame. The side of the door itself, the frame around the doorway and even the door handles (see chapter 4) are all useful yoga props.

Doors make an excellent prop for lengthening the spine and improving posture. Remember that the spine has four natural, gentle curves, but many people over 50 have developed too much rounding of the midback and upper back, and too much of a sway in the lower back. To understand and improve your posture, stand so that your heels press securely against either side of a door. Position your back so you can gently press your spine against the edge of the door, then grasp the top edge of

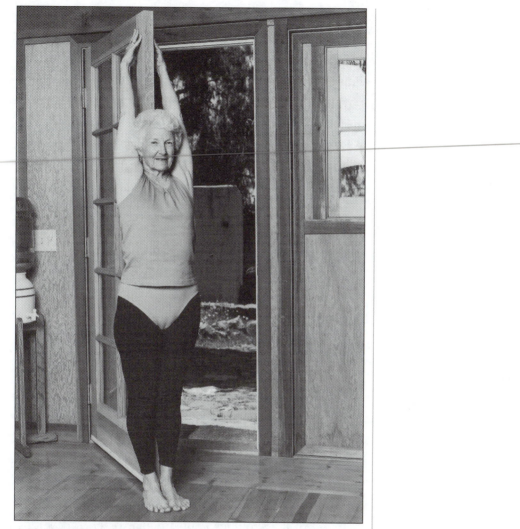

A door can help you discover your true height.

the door as high above your head as you can. The pressure of your back against the door lets you feel your usual alignment and what happens when you stretch upward. The midback may move slightly away from the door while the lower back presses toward the door. Gently draw your navel back toward your spine as you stretch upward and make yourself taller and taller.

This door stretch is also an excellent exercise for removing stiffness in the shoulder joints. In many older people the shoulders are so stiff that when they stretch their arms above their head or try to stretch up the doorway, their elbows bend. With regular practice, shoulders stretch and arms straighten.

Depending on the design of the door or doorway, this exercise can also be done in the doorway itself (taller people will get a better stretch in the doorway). Line up your spine with the center of the doorway and follow the directions for lengthening the spine. As your shoulders regain their natural flexibility, walk your hands farther back, while gently drawing your navel back toward your spine to avoid over-arching or swaying your back.

Stretching Stiff Shoulders with Straps or Belts

To avoid pulled muscles, overstretching and joint strain, never force or rush your body into a yoga position. Use straps and belts, instead, to help you achieve a healthier, more balanced stretch.

The following shoulder stretch, known in Sanskrit as *Gomukhasana* or Cow Face Pose, works on the muscles that control the shoulder joint. Regular practice develops greater freedom of movement so that rounded shoulders can return to healthy posture. If you cannot clasp your hands together, use a strap as a bridge between your two hands as illustrated. This shoulder rotator exercise is one of the most basic corrective poses for removing stiffness from the shoulder joints (the collarbones at the front, arm bones and shoulder blades at the back). It is especially valuable for those who play tennis and other racket sports.

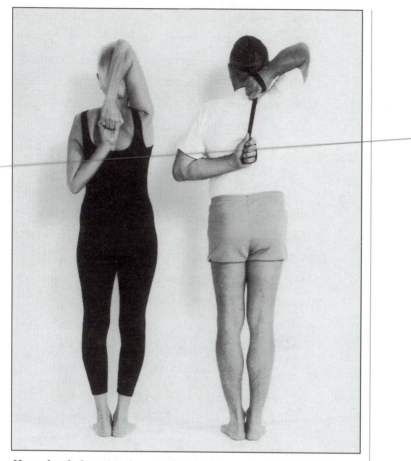

If your hands do not touch, use a strap to help you stretch your shoulders.

Shoulder Stretch Practice

1. Stand (or sit) in your best, tallest posture. Pause for a moment to observe your breath. Allow yourself to smile. This will naturally relax your jaw and face muscles.
2. Stretch your right arm straight up over your head and then bend your elbow so that your palm touches your back between the shoulder blades. Reach across with your left hand to move your elbow closer to your head.

3. Release your left hand from your right elbow and bring your left arm straight back behind your body. Bend the left elbow, placing your hand in the middle of your back above your waist, palm out. Without distorting your posture or straining, try to clasp your hands together as illustrated by the teacher on the left.

4. If your fingers just barely touch, or if there is a big space between your hands, hold a strap or sock in your right hand and gradually work your hands together. Stretch up through the top elbow and down through the bottom elbow. Keep your head centered, face relaxed. Hold at least half a minute. Repeat on the left side. Learn from your more flexible side and repeat or hold longer on the tighter side.

Stretching Stiff Leg Muscles with Straps or Belts

A strap, towel or soft belt around your feet while lying on the floor helps your spine to remain long and stable. Using a strap allows you to gradually stretch and lengthen stiff leg muscles without straining your back.

Lying-Down Leg Stretch with a Strap

1. Lie on your back with your knees bent, feet flat on the floor. If your head tilts back with your chin higher then your forehead, place a folded blanket under your head and neck. Check to see that your upper body is in line with your legs. Allow your back to relax into the floor.

2. Bend your right knee in toward your chest and wrap a strap, towel, soft belt or necktie around the

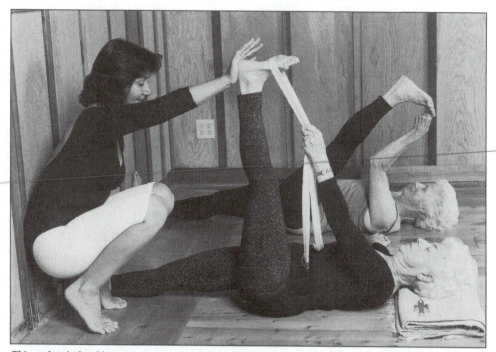

This student in her 80s uses a strap to stretch her legs while the more experienced student next to her practices the Lying Down Big Toe Pose.

ball of your foot. Hold the strap with your right hand. Stretch your left arm out in line with your shoulder on the floor, palm facing up.

3. Slowly straighten your right leg and stretch your toes toward your face. Walk your hand higher up the strap, toward your foot, till your arm is straight. Keep your shoulders and rest of your back relaxed on the floor.

4. If your right hand is quite far away from your foot, keep your left knee bent. If you find it easy to hold your big toe, or if your right hand is high up the strap close to your foot, you can deepen the stretch by practicing this pose with the bottom leg straight, extending through both heels, as illustrated. Stretch your toes toward your face to lengthen your calves and Achilles tendons.

5. Smile and allow your face muscles to relax. Let your breath flow freely, stretching deeper as you exhale. Hold the strap firmly without creating tension in your hand. Enjoy the feeling of the back of your leg lengthening. Hold for about half a minute, longer as you learn to relax and cooperate with the pose. Repeat on the opposite side. If you are practicing with both legs straight, it is helpful to extend the lower heel into the wall.

Improving Your Posture and Breathing Using Bolsters and Blankets

Bolsters, folded blankets and towels are used to support the back of the body in various lying-down positions. Placed along the length of the spinal column and back of the head, these props help correct poor postural and breathing habits, which are often magnified after age 50. The shape of the blanket or pillow supports and encourages the natural curves of the spine. Supported lying-down positions open and expand the chest to improve your posture and breathing.

Most people respond with a delightful sigh of relief when they are positioned on the folded blankets or firm pillows. I consider the use of these props absolutely essential in a yoga program for people over 50.

Because the body tends to sink and collapse into soft materials such as thermal or fluffy blankets, quilts, comforters, sleeping bags or soft pillows, these do not work as yoga props. Heavy cotton or wool blankets that form a firm pad when folded, or bolsters (both of which can be ordered from the addresses in the Resources section or are available through your local yoga center) are best for practicing yoga postures.

The *pranayama,* or breathing bolster, is firm and narrow and supports your spinal column from the lower back to your head when you are lying down. By supporting your spine and opening and expanding the chest, the muscles of your abdomen, chest and back release their tension, lengthen and relax deeply. This bolster is specifically designed so that the sides of your rib cage open and expand over the bolster and move downward toward the floor. When your rib cage expands laterally in this manner, your breathing capacity naturally deepens. The bolster leaves a lasting vital impression on the body of what it feels like to have the chest open and free. Using it enhances your awareness of the breath and your ability to regulate and deepen both your inhalations and exhalations by encouraging you to relax.

You can achieve a similar effect using two or three firm blankets, folded lengthwise.

How to Use a Bolster or Folded Blanket to Relax

1. Sit on the floor with your bolster or folded blankets behind you—the edge of the bolster touching your lower spine, and its length extending behind you. (Your bottom should be completely off the bolster.) Place one or two neatly folded blankets at the other end of the bolster to support your head. Look to see that you are centered with the bolster or blankets.

2. Lower your body backwards, supporting your weight on your elbows, so that your back and head rest on the bolster.

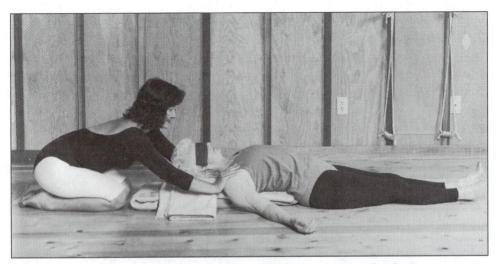

Lying back on blankets or bolsters opens your chest and allows your breath to flow freely.

3. Before lying all the way down, look down the front of your body and see if your chin is in line with the center of your chest, navel and pubic bone. If necessary, adjust the position of your torso so that the straight line formed by your nose, chin, center of your chest, navel and pubic bone extends directly toward a center point between your heels.

4. Continue lowering your spine slowly on the bolster or blankets, without shifting your torso to the left or the right. Before resting the back of your head on the bolster or folded blanket, tuck the additional folded blanket under your head, to bring your forehead slightly higher than your chin. Your forehead should not drop back.

This relaxing position can be practiced with the legs extended, as illustrated, or with a rolled blanket under the knees. Your body should feel supremely comfortable, supported by the bolster, blankets and the floor. (See chapter 12 for more information on the art of conscious relaxation.)

Covering Your Eyes Enhances Relaxation

Placing an eyebag over your eyes will help you relax. An eye covering helps quiet the mind by creating darkness and removing visual stimuli, by relaxing the muscles around your eyes and by calming the involuntary movements of your eyes. After you become familiar with placing your body on the bolster or folded blanket, hold the eye covering in both hands. Eyebags are usually filled with seeds or rice, so distribute the contents evenly. Place the eyebag over your closed eyelids. The eyebag's gentle pressure should feel soothing. Once you've positioned the eyebag, relax your arms on the floor with your hands about a foot away from your hips. Turn your palms up and stretch your fingers outward, turning your thumbs toward the floor. Let your hands soften and relax. (See photo on previous page.)

If an eyebag is not available, use a folded damp washcloth or similar material, placed neatly like a band over your eyes. Eyebags are easy to make by sewing cotton or soft, silky fabric into an 8- or 10-inch bag, about 3½-inches wide (to cover eyes but not nose), filled with about 8 ounces of rice or flax seeds. Or you can even fill a soft cotton sock with rice or flax seed and sew up one end.

Props to Relieve Stress on the Head and Neck

Certain yoga postures such as Headstand or Shoulderstand put unaccustomed weight on the head, neck and shoulders. Yoga props are available to relieve the stress of weight-bearing by supporting most or all of

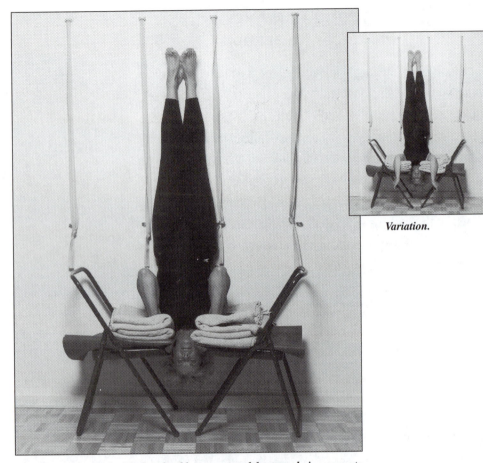

Variation.

Headstand practiced with the shoulders supported by two chairs prevents neck strain and allows beginners or people with neck problems to practice without injuring the neck.

your body weight as you practice these poses. A prop known as the Headstander, for example, supports nearly 90 percent of your weight, enabling you to practice the Headstand without bearing weight on your neck. Similarly, the Halasana bench supports most of your weight and frees your neck as you practice Shoulder-stand and Plow Pose. Both of these props are available through the sources listed in the Resources section. (Refer to chapter 11 on Restful Inversions.)

The Backbending Bench

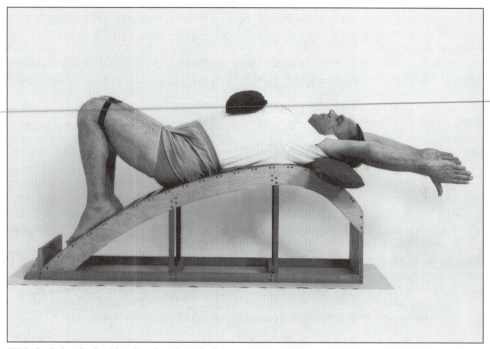

With the help of a backbending bench and other yoga props, older students can safely experience the rejuvenating effects of a backbend.

Yoga postures give a sense of delight, lightness, buoyancy, vitality, balance and health. When our muscles are too tight or weak, or we are afraid of putting our bodies in positions or shapes that they have not been in for many years, props are a way of removing the obstacles between you and a pose that seems out of reach. With a backbending bench, available for use at many yoga centers, almost anyone can begin to practice a safe, supported backbend. This bench supports and lengthens your spine, stretches your arms and shoulders, opens your rib cage and lungs, deepens your breathing, stretches your groin, abdomen and the front of your thighs.

Lying on the backbending bench presses the vertebrae of your upper back toward the center of your body. This movement opens your chest and counteracts the rounding of the upper back.

My older students especially enjoy and benefit from lying on this bench. If you have neck or back problems, learn to use the backbending bench with the help of a qualified instructor, as you may need extra support under your head, neck or back.

Back and Neck Pain

Yoga differs from other types of rehabilitative exercise in that it engages the whole person. Yoga-based relaxation techniques and stretching and strengthening exercises are effective because the mind is focused in a meditative way on your movements, skin and muscle sensations, and relaxed breathing. Mind and body work together, creating a physiological and psychological environment that optimizes the potential for healing.
—*Mary Pullig Schatz, M.D., Back Care Basics: A Doctor's Gentle Yoga Program for Back and Neck Pain Relief*

People with back and neck pain generally experience relief practicing yoga, with the help of the props presented in this chapter. For in-depth instruction on how yoga can relieve back and neck pain, I highly recommend the guidance offered in the book, *Back Care Basics: A Doctor's Gentle Yoga Program for Back and Neck Pain Relief*, by Mary Pullig Schatz, M.D.

In addition to a gentle yoga program, other therapeutic techniques such as chiropractic and massage can be helpful. Many people with back and neck problems experience both temporary and long-term relief from chiropractic adjustments. A chiropractor familiar with yoga is ideal. Yoga will allow you to progress beyond symptomatic relief by correcting the weaknesses and misalignments in your body, changing your postural habits, and teaching you to relax and cope constructively with stress.

Exercising After Back Injury or Surgery

When the back or neck hurts, it is instinctive to seek relief from pain by resting and avoiding further strain.

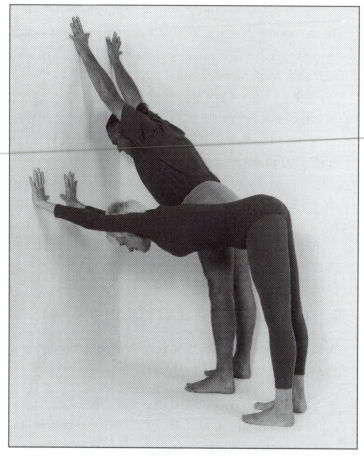

Standing poses like this Forward Stretch with Hands High on the Wall help to keep your back healthy for a lifetime.

People with back problems often fear that any movement or exercise might cause re-injury. But without an intelligent exercise program that addresses the underlying causes of back pain—unhealthy posture, muscles that are too tight or weak and poor body mechanics in daily life—re-injury is practically inevitable.

If the body remains immobilized beyond a reasonable period of rest, the muscles that support the back become weaker and increasingly vulnerable to re-injury. To break the cycle of further deterioration, inactivity and pain, we need to learn how to practice yoga, and which type of exercise rehabilitates our back and which type of exercise or yoga practice hurts it.

Dr. Schatz points out that some people feel so good after surgery or in between "back attacks" that they mistakenly imagine that their injuries have healed. Without pain as a reminder, the need to care for the back tends to recede in our consciousness. However, if surgery has taken place, post-surgical structural weaknesses and muscular weakness, aggravated by prolonged bed rest and combined with underlying problems contribute to the likelihood of more back problems in the future.

B.K.S. Iyengar On Using Props

B.K.S. Iyengar asserts that very few people make use of the last phase of life in a fruitful way.

It is an art to check the aging process. To stop its ascendance, one should learn to make old age a useful weapon. In this stage of life, one becomes negative. Courage starts declining and intelligence becomes dull. Anxiety encircles the older person. Laziness becomes a part of old age.

Some in old age realize the importance of yoga and come for help. They have not done any yogic practice before and want to learn and do something; yet they are unable to do the yoga postures. At that state, the profound utility of props and their values are realized. Even incapable persons will find hope of doing something that keeps life flowing with joy.

Iyengar believes that students who come to yoga late in life get the advantage of keeping themselves fit physically and mentally using props. His experience has been that bolsters, backbending and other benches, ropes and other props are useful in old age, when people may not be able to do the posture independently. He believes that props free the older student from anxiety. "Practice on props leads one toward non-attachment of the body. The brain calms down and sound sleep, a dream for many old people, comes naturally through the use of props," says Iyengar.

More ways to use yoga props are explained throughout this book.

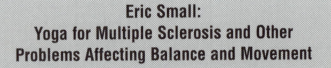

Eric Small:
Yoga for Multiple Sclerosis and Other
Problems Affecting Balance and Movement

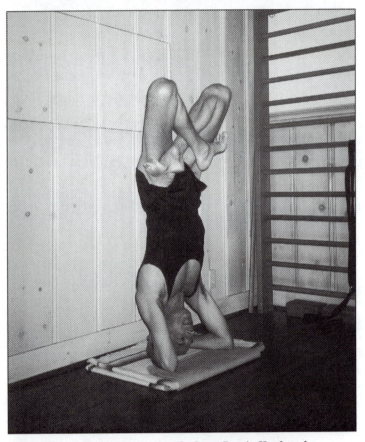

Eric Small, in his 60s, demonstrates the Lotus Pose in Headstand.

Eric Small, a Los Angeles yoga teacher in his 60s, keeps multiple sclerosis in remission by practicing yoga.

Multiple sclerosis (MS) is a disease that prevents proper functioning of the body's electrical circuitry. It attacks the insulation (the myelin sheath) around the electrical wiring (the nerves) of the body, causing the myelin sheath to unravel and deteriorate, leaving behind gaps and scar tissue. Consequently, electrical signals do not flow effectively along the nerve pathways, and the system short-circuits. Symptoms of MS include loss of balance, loss of sight, speech impairment, organ dysfunction, motor impairment, numbness, pain and loss of energy. Stress and/or fatigue can severely exacerbate these conditions.

Over 40 years ago I found that my body was no longer responding to signals my brain sent it. I felt like a telephone that always dialed a wrong number, got a busy signal, or found no one at home. The diagnosis: MS.

After I was diagnosed with MS, I underwent every known therapy at the time. Then I discovered hatha yoga. At first the discipline was very hard to come to. As I gained confidence and stopped falling down so much, I started to respond to yoga and gained strength and flexibility. My nervous system was relieved of stress. Little by little, I learned to use my mind to communicate with non-responsive areas in my body. Sometimes I even developed alternative solutions to execute normal functions.

I found that by using props, I could maintain the *asanas* (yoga postures) better. One of the most important tools was water. In the buoyancy of the pool, gravity and muscle strength were no longer negative factors. The water was also very relaxing, and helped moderate my body temperature. (Overheating is a "no-no" for anyone with MS).

When I took my first Iyengar-style class, bells went off. The alignment, the concentration and, of course, the props were exciting and effective. I still use many props in my own daily practice, as well as when I teach yoga to other people who have MS. I find that the Iyengar system allows the MS student to achieve the beneficial effects of the asanas without too much frustration or fatigue.

I have been teaching hatha yoga to other MS students for many years, and find the best place to start is with the breath, to set aside time both in and out of class to develop a smooth breathing pattern. This helps students to calm down and center themselves. It also soothes the nervous system. Working with this general breathing pattern is time well spent. It builds a confidence that the MS student carries into the adventure of learning asanas.

Each case of MS is unique. The symptoms, the degree of nerve degradation, and thus the general health of each individual can vary tremendously. It is of vital importance to ascertain each student's abilities to discover which asanas are most important. The key to asanas for the MS student is to be gentle, not over-ambitious. No pose should be held too long, as this causes fatigue and overheating. Poses need to be supported in whatever way possible to accomplish this. I use walls, chairs, belts, benches, pillows, bolsters, the horse, and even lie flat on the floor for certain poses.

For MS students who use wheelchairs, I have developed an amazing series of asanas that require a folding chair and a belt. Some of my students have even been able to get up into supported Shoulderstand with my help. Though they may still need it, bit by bit these students become less dependent on the wheelchair. Then their whole attitude toward themselves and life improves.

Although hatha yoga is not a cure for MS, it can slow some of its negative effects. I have seen so many positive results over the years: increased blood circulation, improvement in digestive and eliminative processes, more effective muscle performance and increased security in balance, among others. Yoga improves the use of secondary and alternative ways for the body to function. Self-esteem and confidence increase. Students learn to incorporate the knowledge and skills developed through the practice of yoga into their everyday lives. This reduces stress and fatigue, and dramatically improves their lives. Using yoga techniques, I have remained symptom-free.

We make a disclaimer that yoga will not cure MS, but that it is a way of teaching the physically limited. I get people out of a wheelchair and into a regular chair right away—by the second or third class, often the first. One man came in like a crab, as if he were palsied instead of suffering from MS—all contorted in on himself and angry. Now he smiles. His feet and legs were all swollen. Now they're normal. He now sits on a regular chair and gets on the floor to do Shoulderstands, with help. Another man was 84 when he first came to me. He didn't have MS, he was an old man dying. His leg was blue-black from lack of circulation. In three months he had a pink and healthy leg. This man just turned 90.

Hatha yoga is effective where physical therapy isn't, in that you become your own teacher. In yoga, one's breath, mind and body work together to control physical movement.

Four

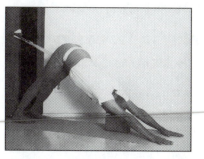

Key Yoga Postures for Reversing the Aging Process

In the mornings, Monday through Friday, we do our yoga exercises. I started doing yoga exercises with Mama about 40 years ago. Mama was starting to shrink up and get bent down, and I started exercising with her to straighten her up again. . . . When Bessie turned 80 she decided that I looked better than her so she decided she would start doing yoga too . . .

—Sarah and Elizabeth Delany, at ages 102 and 104,
authors of *Having Our Say, the Delany Sister's First 100 Years*

Downward- and Upward-Facing Dog Pose

Adho Mukha Svanasana and *Urdhva Mukha Svanasana*

The Downward-Facing Dog Pose is named for the way dogs instinctively stretch their bodies. When practiced with the hands on the floor, the shape of the pose resembles a dog stretching, with the arms and hands stretched out like a dog's forepaws, the shoulders, spine and chest stretching and the pelvis and tailbone high, stretching back away from the hands. When dogs stretch they do so with great enjoyment—with all their heart and soul. Naturally, we humans should stretch in a similar way.

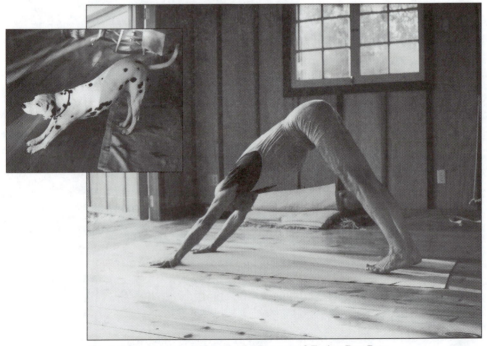

Frank White enjoys stretching in the Downward-Facing Dog Pose.

A panacea for people over 50, this ingenious whole-body stretching and strengthening pose combines the benefits of going upside down and bending forward. It is actually like an entire yoga session rolled into one. My experience has been that even octogenarians who may not have stretched for many years—and who may initially have trouble kneeling and getting down and back up from the floor—can begin to enjoy this pose very early in their practice.

Many of my students who started yoga in their 70s or 80s could barely go back and forth from Downward- to Upward-Facing Dog once before their arms collapsed. Now these same experienced students enjoy practicing Upward- and Downward-Facing Dog 10 times or more, both with a chair (as illustrated on the next page) and from the floor.

Downward-Facing Dog Pose is a halfway inverted position that almost everyone can safely practice. This pose inverts the internal organs and increases blood flow to the head. A weight-bearing pose, it strengthens the hands, wrists, arms and shoulders and stimulates bones to retain calcium, thus helping to prevent osteoporosis. Downward- and Upward-Facing Dog poses work together to remove a lifetime of stiffness from the shoulder joints, wrists, hands and fingers. The whole spinal column is lengthened, abdominal muscles are strengthened and neck tension is released. This pose helps prevent and decrease the roundness of the upper back so common among older people in our culture. It corrects rounded shoulders by stretching the pectoral muscles on the front of the chest and eradicates the obstacles to good posture.

Older students often report that they regain lost height

> Those who are afraid to do Headstand *(Sirsasana)* can conveniently practice this position. As the trunk is lowered in this posture (asana) it is fully stretched and healthy blood is brought to this region without any strain on the heart. It rejuvenates the brain cells and invigorates the brain by relieving fatigue. Persons suffering with high blood pressure can do this pose.
> —*B.K.S. Iyengar,*
> Light on Yoga

after consistently practicing the Downward-Facing Dog and other yoga poses. My students of all ages practice it almost every class, from the floor and with a chair or hanging from ropes or straps.

When practiced from the floor, the Dog Poses require a fair amount of flexibility in the back of the legs, and strength and flexibility in the wrists, arms and shoulders. You can prepare your body by first practicing with the hands on the seat of a chair.

Downward-Facing Dog Pose with a Chair

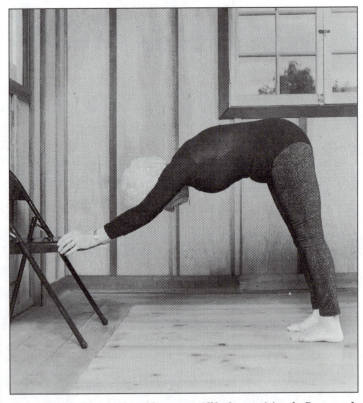

For people who have back problems or a stiff body, practicing the Downward-Facing Dog Pose with a Chair can help you stretch in a healthy way.

1. Put a sturdy, level chair against a wall. Place your hands shoulder-width apart on the front edge of the chair seat. Keeping your hands on the chair, take a giant step back until you are a full arm's-length away, your heels slightly behind your hips, feet hip-width apart.

2. Press your hands firmly into the chair seat and come up high on your toes, lifting your bottom as high up as possible. Stay up on your toes for several breaths as you push the chair away from you and lengthen your spinal column. Push the chair toward the wall, stretch your fingertips as far away as possible and your buttock bones as far back as possible to lengthen your spine to the maximum. Continue pushing the chair away as you slowly lower your heels to the floor. While you press your heels firmly down, pick up all 10 toes and spread them wide apart until you can see daylight between them! Breathe calmly and freely. Smile so that your face muscles relax.

3. To come out of the pose, bring your body forward toward the chair, bend one knee, and stand up, nice and tall. Sit down in the chair for a few moments if you feel light-headed or need to rest.

Upward-Facing Dog Pose with a Chair

1. Begin in Downward-Facing Dog with hands on the chair seat. To move into Upward-Facing Dog, change the positioning of your hands slightly so that they firmly grip the edges of the chair seat.

2. Keeping your hands firmly gripping the seat of the chair, bring the tops of your thighs and pubic bone

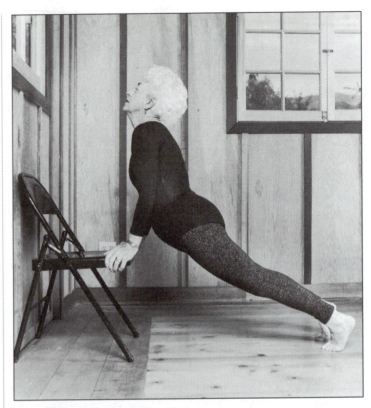

Upward-Facing Dog Pose with a Chair

toward the chair. Continue firmly pressing down into the chair seat, straightening your arms, rolling your shoulders back, lifting your sternum and opening your chest. Look up by taking your head gently back, without constricting your neck.

3. Keep your hands gripping the chair seat as you stretch back into Dog Pose. If you feel unusual strain in your wrists, try padding the chair with a folded sticky mat. As your strength improves, repeat Upward- and Downward-Facing Dog several times. To come out of the pose bring your body forward from Downward Dog back toward the chair, bend one knee and stand up slowly. Sit

down in the chair for a few moments if you feel light-headed or need to rest.

Note: Be careful not to hold your breath. Keep your breath flowing. Stay in the Upward and Downward Dog Poses long enough so you feel your body strengthening and lengthening, but not so long that your arms collapse. Observe the positioning of your toes as you move from Downward into Upward Dog. As your thighs move closer to the chair, you will feel your toes turning.

Downward-Facing Dog Pose from the Floor

1. Kneel on all fours on a non-slippery floor, so that your hands do not slide. Position your knees slightly behind your hips, toes curled under as shown, your feet and knees hip-width (about 18 inches) apart. Place your hands slightly in front of your shoulders, shoulder-distance apart. Spread all

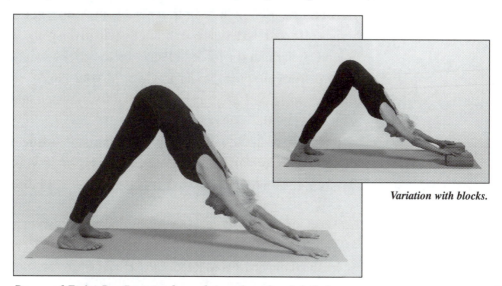

Variation with blocks.

Downward-Facing Dog Pose stretches and strengthens the whole body.

10 fingers wide apart and press both hands down onto the floor.

2. On an exhale, straighten your knees and lift your bottom toward the ceiling, so that your body forms a high upside-down V or pyramid shape. Raise your heels high off the floor and try to lift your bottom higher and higher. Press your hands deep into the floor, as if you are pushing the floor away from you. After stretching for a few breaths with your heels lifted, try pressing your heels down toward the floor, as illustrated on pages 64 and 69.

3. Breathe smoothly, naturally. Keep your face and neck relaxed and soft. Imagine roots pulling your hands and feet into the earth while the top of your buttocks, your tailbone, extends toward the sky. Release, come back to kneeling on all fours. Slowly lower your bottom back toward your heels and lower your torso and forehead to the floor in Child's Pose. (See chapter 6, page 140.)

A common complaint in this pose is pressure on the wrists. If your wrists are extremely sensitive, place a folded sticky mat (or folded blanket on the sticky mat to keep it from slipping) under the heel of your hands, so that the wrist part of your hand is slightly elevated and supported by the extra cushioning.

Do not stay in the pose if your back hurts, if you feel unusual pressure in the head or dizziness, or if your wrists and shoulders ache. Ask a yoga teacher for help.

Upward-Facing Dog Pose

In the Upward-Facing Dog Pose, the body is supported by the hands and feet. The legs and pubic bone

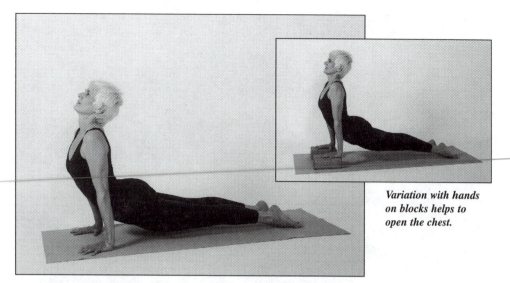

*Variation with hands
on blocks helps to
open the chest.*

Upward-Facing Dog Pose.

are off the floor. Older beginners generally find it easier
to practice the pose by shifting their weight forward and
then lowering their body into Upward-Facing Dog Pose.

1. Lie face down on a non-slippery surface. Position
   your hands next to your chest, keeping your elbows
   close to your body. Place your feet hip-width apart.
   Stretch your legs back and pull your kneecaps up
   so that your thigh muscles feel firm.
2. On an inhalation, lift your upper body off the floor,
   straightening your arms. Lift and open your chest.
   Look forward or slightly up, keeping your neck
   long and relaxed, your shoulders stretching back
   and down. Try to bring your legs and pubic bone off
   the floor. Keep your buttock muscles firm and your
   legs stretching back. Press down with your hands,
   straighten the arms more and lift your trunk away
   from the floor. Keep breathing! Do not sink the
   weight of your body toward the floor.

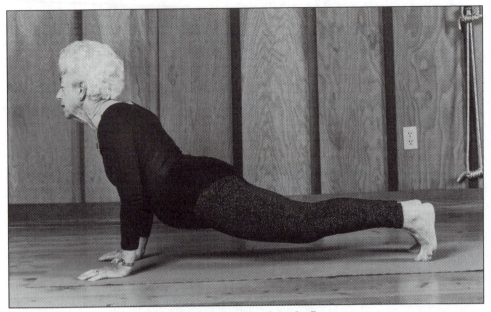

A student in her 80s practices Upward-Facing Dog Pose from the floor.

Lower yourself to the floor and relax in Child's Pose.

As strength improves, stretch from Upward-Facing Dog back into Downward-Facing Dog. Rest by bending your knees back to the floor and relax in Child's Pose.

The human body contains approximately 650 muscles, all imprinted with the same ageless message: Use it or lose it. Downward- and Upward-Facing Dog poses develop the strength and shape of long-forgotten muscles and stimulate bone growth, preventing brittle bones and osteoporosis. Most problems in these poses can be overcome by experimenting on your own or with the help of a qualified teacher.

Other Variations of Downward-Facing Dog: Downward-Facing Dog Hanging from a Rope or Strap

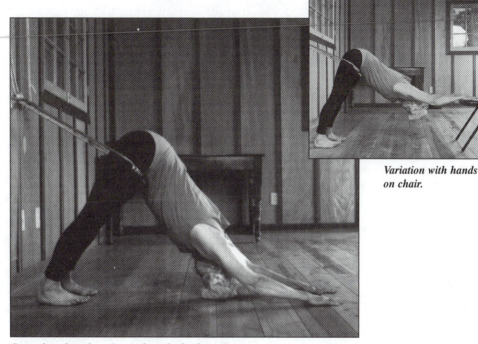

Variation with hands on chair.

Ropes lengthen the spine and soothe back tension.

In Downward-Facing Dog Hanging from a Rope, the rope supports most of your weight, allowing you to let go and lengthen your body even more. Hanging from a rope allows you to hold the pose longer, thereby giving the back of the body a deeper stretch. The gentle traction of this pose eases many types of back pain, tension or spasm, while at the same time restoring the natural, youthful curves of the spine.

For people who come to yoga with a rounded back, Dog Pose Hanging from a Rope is invaluable, especially followed by a session with wall ropes going back and forth. You can purchase professional yoga wall ropes from the prop sources listed in the back of this book. Or make a loop out of a strap or soft rope, looped securely over a doorknob or through an eye hook securely attached to a wall stud. Various types of ropes or straps will serve the purpose, but a soft, unbreakable cotton rope or mountain-climbing webbing about six to seven feet long works best. If the strap or rope cuts into your legs, it may not be wide enough. Try either a loop made out of different material, or use a thick towel or smooth blanket to pad the strap if it cuts into your legs.

Look at the photos on pages 75 and 76 and follow these directions carefully.

1. Hook the rope or strap securely around both sides of a sturdy doorknob (the doorknob must be sturdy enough to hold your weight).
2. Step into the loop and place it at the crease at the top of your legs—right where your hips bend at the groin.
3. Lean forward into the rope until your weight feels supported and place your hands on the chair for stability. Make sure the rope is taut—the trick in the beginning is to walk the feet backward while stretching the arms farther forward so that the rope remains taut and does not slip down the legs.
4. Step your feet backwards as you stretch your hands out in front of you on the chair. When you feel secure, move the chair farther away from you, but still keep your hands on the chair.
5. More flexible people can take their hands all the way to the floor so that the body forms an upside-down V

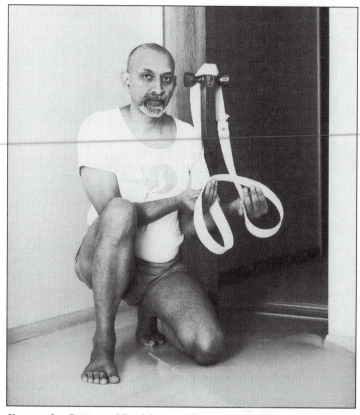

Yoga teacher Ramanand Patel demonstrates how you can hang from a single strap placed at the tops of your legs or with two loops as shown here.

or pyramid. If you find yourself bending your knees to relieve pain in the hamstrings, then place your hands back on the chair. Don't hurry. Eventually you will enjoy stretching in the pose with your hands on the floor.

6. To further lengthen your spine, continue to walk your hands farther away on the chair seat or floor. Keep your legs actively stretching back toward the door behind you, heels stretching down. Feel your spine lengthening (from the top of your tailbone down to the top of your head). Increase the stretch

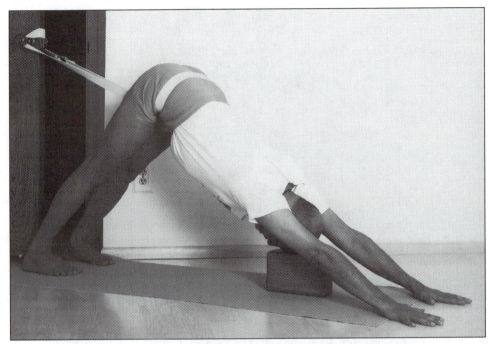

Downward-Facing Dog Pose, with rope around a door knob and a block under the head.

by lifting all 10 toes up off the floor and spreading them wide apart.

7. Hang like this for several breaths, gradually increasing the length of time to about three minutes. Keep your leg muscles active by stretching your heels to the floor and periodically lifting and spreading your toes.

8. To come out, bend your knees and walk your feet toward your hands. As you become more confident and flexible, you can hang forward a little longer with your heels more underneath your hips. If your legs are stiff or your back feels strain, place your hands on a chair.

9. Stand back up on an inhalation. Step back and lean your body back into the wall or door. Stand quietly and notice how you feel.

Restful Downward-Facing Dog with Chair Variation

Instead of lowering your palms to the chair or floor, clasp each elbow in the opposite hand and rest the elbows on the seat of the chair, lengthening your upper body as much as possible. Rest your forehead on your forearms, or place a bolster, stack of folded blankets or towels on the seat of the chair. If you're still uncomfortable and unable to lengthen your spine, turn the chair around and rest your head on your forearms on the back of the chair.

Cautions for Downward Dog Pose Hanging from a Rope or Strap

Be sure to practice on a non-slippery surface without socks. Be careful not to lose your balance as you step in and out of the rope. If you tend to feel dizzy or light-headed after forward-bending poses, stay in them for shorter periods and increase the time gradually. If you feel unsteady, practice with a sturdy chair within reach. Hanging from ropes secured to a wall makes the pose more stable; plus, you can lean back into the wall when you step out of the rope.

Yoga Master B.K.S. Iyengar designed this way of practicing the Downward-Facing Dog Pose. At his institute in India and yoga centers all over the world, the ropes are attached to hooks in the wall, as illustrated on page 73.

Right-Angle Handstand with a Wall or Other Yoga Prop

Turn page 57 sideways to view Right-Angle Handstand from an upright position. Note that if you

were upside down stretching at the wall, your hands
would be on the floor, and your feet on the wall approximately at the height where your hands are when you
are standing upright. To prepare for Right-Angle
Handstand, practice stretching with your hands flat on
the wall, shoulder distance apart, feet hip-width apart,
your body approximately at a right angle (see page 57).

If you are unsure of your upper body strength, I recommend you first learn Right-Angle Handstand with the
help of a teacher before practicing on your own. Some
yoga centers have a prop called the "horse," a braced
wooden frame similar to the trestle used in gymnastics.
This yoga prop is extremely useful for learning the
dynamics of Right-Angle Handstand and other important poses.

Before proceeding, review the cautions on inverted
poses in chapters 2 and 11.

Right-Angle Handstand is a good example of how
yoga strengthens your upper body without sacrificing
flexibility. As I mentioned in the introduction, this pose
requires quite a bit of strength and daring. Regularly
stretching with your hands on a wall, and practicing the
Downward- and Upward-Facing Dog Poses, will give
you the strength and flexibility you need to safely practice this Upside-Down Pose.

How to Practice
Right-Angle Handstand

1. Practice Right-Angle Handstand by positioning
   your body as if you are doing the Downward-
   Facing Dog with your heels on the wall. Kneel on
   the floor, place your hands about four feet away

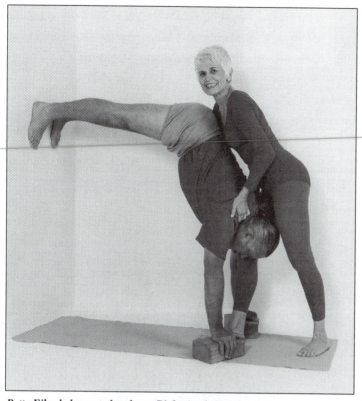

Betty Eiler helps a student learn Right-Angle Handstand.

from the wall, shoulder distance apart, and come up into Dog Pose with heels secure on the baseboard.

2. When you feel ready, walk your feet up the wall in a backward Handstand until they are as high (or a little higher) than your hips, forming a right angle as illustrated. Hold as long as your arms feel strong and secure. Walk down the wall. Move your bottom back toward your heels and lower your torso and forehead to the floor (Child's Pose).

If your wrists feel sensitive, place a folded sticky mat, a wedge or a block (made for this purpose, available at most yoga centers) under the heel of your hands as illustrated, so that the wrist part of your hand is slightly elevated and supported by the extra lift. Be sure to place any extra support for your hands on a non-slippery sticky mat.

Handstand in the Hallway or Doorway

Handstands are also known as Full Arm Balance or *Adho Mukha Vrksasana*—meaning Upside-Down Tree Pose in Sanskrit.

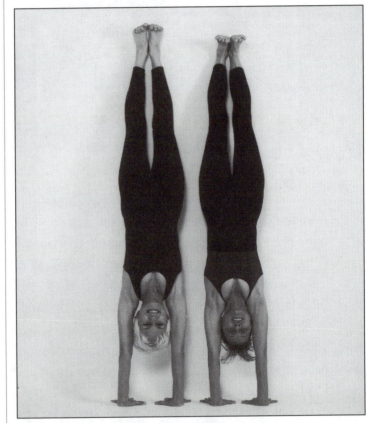

Full Arm Balance is energizing and strengthening.

For me as a teacher, it is especially fun and rewarding to help students over 50 learn to kick up into Handstands with confidence. Whenever I feel lethargic or grumpy, I find a wall or a tree and kick up into a Handstand. This pose immediately changes your perspective and you feel like a kid again. If you are a grandparent, you can experience the thrill of your grandchild proudly bringing you to school to demonstrate Handstands in front of the whole class for "show and tell"— as several of my students have reported.

A hallway or doorway is an excellent prop for students who don't have enough momentum or confidence to kick up into a Handstand. Start by practicing the Right-Angle Handstand in a hallway. Start in Downward-Facing Dog with your heels on the wall. Walk the feet up the wall behind you as high as you can. While one foot secures the position by pressing into the wall, the other leg swings up to the vertical position, bringing you into a Handstand. A wide doorway can be used in a similar way.

For safety's sake, be sure to have an experienced teacher guide you the first few times you try this. Your teacher can help you establish the right distance for your hands from the wall or door frame. The exact distance you place your hands from the wall depends on your height, flexibility and the size of the hall or doorway.

Ruth Barati:
Feeling Vital and Vibrant in Your 70s

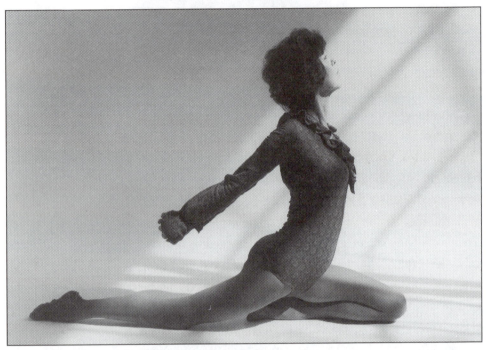

This pose shows the strength and grace that is the heart of yoga.

For over 40 years, yoga has been my constant companion, my source, my solace, my gateway to joy. What began as a pleasant diversion became a discipline for growth, an ongoing apprenticeship in awareness, attention, mindful observation and commitment.

Its physical, ethical and philosophic foundation allows me in my 70s to wake up each day feeling vital and vibrant, supple and strong, eager to confront the challenges of the world around me and the world within. I continue to delight in the passions of the body and the inquiring journeys of the mind.

Yoga has taught me that the body and mind are partners, not adversaries or strangers to each other, and that there is no paradox in embodied spirituality. This interaction has guided me to a calm center from which I can summon at will serenity and peace, a sense of being part of the mystery and order of the universe and an intuition of union with others. In addition, sharing yoga with my husband and two daughters has given us a refuge and source of strength in adversity and a loving fountain of well-being when the sun has smiled upon us.

The crown has been the humbling and awesome privilege of teaching. The purpose of teaching yoga is for our mutual opening and heart healing. The men and women of all ages (teenagers to people in their 90s) in class journey together into the frontiers of our bodies, minds and spirits. Their insights, wisdom, responsiveness and love are priceless gifts as moment by moment they are teaching me.

The ultimate reward is to watch my students throw off tension and stress and awaken to the messages of the body, as conscious breathing creates a bridge to an enlivened mind and the asanas change their bodies and alter their reality. Divisions within them heal, allowing them to act with wisdom. Centered, they experience in their very tissues a consciousness that makes all that the organism is and does meaningful.

Elizabeth T. Shuey, a student of Ruth Barati

All my life I had been intrigued with yoga, but was never really exposed to it or learned very much about it. That was to change.

After six months on crutches following a hip injury, someone suggested I take a yoga class. As a young person, I had been active in sports, in school and out, was a swimmer and hiker. The long months of living on crutches resulted in stiffness and considerable frustration with my enforced inactivity.

The teacher, Ruth Barati, welcomed me to my first yoga class with such genuine warmth and understanding. She was willing to guide me through activities appropriate to my limited ability. Very soon I realized my upper torso and leg were responding to stretching and relaxation and my spirits were lifted. When I was finally able to bear weight on both legs, she continued to teach and encourage me as I grew stronger. Her quiet and beautiful presence brought a serenity into my life, even when I was grappling with grief over the deaths of both my husband and mother. Ten years later I am still attending her class, and she continues to renew and refresh my spirit and body. I am in better touch with my inner self.

What does yoga mean to me? It means adding a dimension to my life that wasn't there before. When I walk into that room I am aware of a deep spirit, an area of quietness, of loveliness, where there is caring, respect, gentleness; where images and directed thought lead me away from the noise and clutter of the day to an inner awareness of body, mind and spirit.

Yoga has given me a greater respect for the human body and its amazing potential. I am no longer discouraged by its weaknesses, many of which I now see are unconsciously self-induced. Through yoga I have learned the value of stretching and strengthening postures, which have greatly increased my flexibility and feelings of well-being. The awareness of the importance of breathing in its varied forms is a continual theme throughout yoga, the benefits of which are enormous.

I welcome the quiet meditative aspects of yoga, centering myself and the feeling of continuity with the wisdom of ages past. When I am tense and tired and feeling perhaps somewhat older than I'd like to feel, yoga gives me a wonderful feeling of peace, perspective and renewed strength.

Five

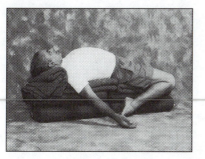

Yoga for Feet and Knees Over 50

Healthy Feet and Knees Can Make the Difference Between Walking and a Wheelchair

Taking up yoga again at age 50, after a hiatus of many years, has been both a revelation and confirmation to me. On the one hand, yoga now has revealed that strength and flexibility can still be mine. On the other hand, somehow I knew that this was true, given my active and healthy lifestyle. As my body increases in flexibility with each week of class, my dedication to the practice increases as well. With the practice comes a new peace of mind through the process of yoga.

—MINDY LORENZ, YOGA STUDENT

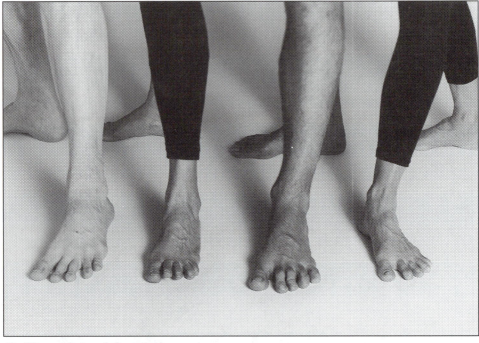

Healthy yoga feet ready for action!

The feet are our foundation. They connect us to the earth. Yet an awareness of the relationship between our feet and the health of the whole body is often literally the farthest thing from our minds. Let's take a fresh look at these two faithful servants that, in the course of a lifetime, will walk an estimated 115,000 miles—the equivalent of four-and-a-half strolls around the planet.

One of the first features that impressed me about my older yoga teachers was their feet. Their toes could spread wide apart like fingers. In contrast, most of the elderly people I took care of had toes so jammed together from a lifetime imprisoned in too-tight shoes that walking was painful. It was practically impossible to clean the spaces between their toes. Their ankles were swollen and dark from poor circulation. I realized that

> You have to learn to listen to your body, going with it and not against it. . . . You will be amazed to discover that, if you are kind to your body, it will respond in an incredible way.
>
> —*Vanda Scaravelli*,
> Awakening the Spine

stretching and strengthening the feet, ankles and toes are absolutely imperative for maintaining one's mobility and independence.

Every architect realizes that the structure of a building depends on a solid foundation for its strength. When the foundation is weak or flawed, problems arise throughout the building. Likewise, many aches and pains—backaches, headaches, leg cramps, even a cranky disposition—can be traced to the body's foundation, the feet. There is a lot of truth to the adage, "When your feet hurt, you hurt all over."

On average, a person takes 10,000 steps every day. Healthy feet are crucial for an active and independent lifestyle, yet four out of five adults experience foot pain—and most of these people are over 50. Surveys indicate that most people think that foot pain is normal. This may be one reason why foot problems that tend to worsen with age are too often ignored.

There are many common ailments of the feet. These include weak, fallen arches; displaced, deformed, overlapping toes; claw toes; hammer toes; calluses and corns; bunions and big toes that seem to be glued to their neighbors. Who or what is the real culprit behind these problems? The shoe industry! Most difficulties people have with their toes and feet are caused or aggravated by shoes that place too much pressure on them. With all the wide, comfortable and attractive shoes available now, it is amazing that shoe manufacturers persist in creating insidious styles that cramp, crowd and squash the feet until the toes are stiff and all but the faintest hint of life has been pressed out of them. Surveys by the University of Southern California School of Medicine and the American Orthopedic Foot

Healing people and healing the planet are part of the same enterprise. People have a deep psychological need for contact with nature; the planet needs the reverential care of humans.

—*Theodore Roszak,*
The Voice of the Earth

and Ankle Society found that 88 percent of women were wearing shoes smaller than their feet and 80 percent complained that their feet hurt.

If the shoe industry stopped manufacturing their tight, narrow, toe-crunching products, we would not lose the spaces between our toes that we had as young children. I am an unabashed fanatic when it comes to wearing shoes that are big enough to spread all 10 toes, just as if I were barefoot. I also find that most people actually believe that their shoes have plenty of room, but the shape of their feet from a lifetime jammed in cramped quarters tells a different story.

The 26 bones of the feet need ample space to distribute and balance the weight of the body. You may not think your shoes are too tight, but if you cannot spread all 10 toes wide apart, then your feet need wider shoes, more time barefoot and yoga. Lack of space results in the over-use or under-use of bones, muscles, tendons and ligaments, and the entire body must compensate. High heels throw off the ankles, knees and hips, the sacroiliac joint, the lower and upper back, the neck, and may even affect the jaw.

If you figure that your parents probably put you in shoes prematurely—often before you began walking—then add the years of adulthood in closed shoes, it is no wonder that feet begin to lose their resilience quite early in life, whether you are athletic or sedentary. Aching feet are one of the first reasons that many older people stop walking—just at a time in their life when the body most needs some healthy, stimulating exercise.

Left untreated, foot ailments alter our body mechanics. Our whole posture is affected by foot problems, which can gradually progress to pain in the ankles, knees, hips, back, and neck and head. Counteracting the effects of aging on the feet requires more than proper hygiene and visits to a local podiatrist. The feet need regular stretching and strengthening exercise such as you experience in yoga.

When I ask my beginning yoga students to lift and stretch all 10 toes wide apart until you can see daylight between them, they usually look at me with utter disbelief. However, as one of my teachers, Mary Dunn, proclaims, "The ability to stretch our toes like fingers and to create a wide, healthy, open space between each and every toe is not some vestigial ability available only to a chosen few."

Revitalizing and Stretching Your Feet

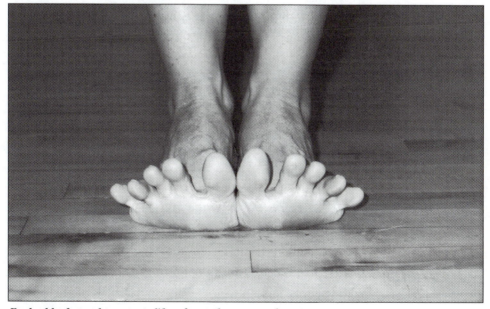

For healthy feet and toes, try to lift and spread your toes whenever you can.

One of the best ways to strengthen your feet is to walk barefoot on natural terrain, just as our ancestors did for the first million years of human history. The more uncomfortable walking barefoot is for you, the more you probably need it! Use common sense. If your feet are very sensitive, start on a smoother, grassy or sandy surface. Then as your feet toughen up, walk on more uneven, pebbly or rocky terrain. This gives the feet a stimulating natural foot massage. (Creek beds are great for this, plus you can slosh through mud or ice cold water, which is very invigorating!)

I'm going to give you the same advice that I give myself: Unless I'm hiking, biking or running, my feet are either bare (in socks around the house on cold days) or in open-toed, comfortable sandal-type shoes. Any chiropractor or podiatrist will be glad to write you a doctor's excuse should your job require heels. The healthier your feet become, the less they will tolerate being crammed into unhealthy shoes.

The combination of walking and yoga is the supreme way to rehabilitate your feet. Walking (in wide shoes, of course!) maintains the overall health of the foot—improves circulation and encourages bone and muscle development as well as improves strength and flexibility in the supporting muscles of the shins, calves and quadriceps.

Try to spread your toes wide apart like fingers. If necessary, reach down with your hands and try to make your two big toes touch each other, as illustrated. Stretch all your toes as far apart as possible; separate the little toe away from its neighbor especially. If your big toe seems unable to move independently of the second toe, pull your toes apart with your fingers every chance you have and practice the toe stretching exercises described on the following pages. Stretching the two big toes toward each other and the little toes away from each other strengthens and lifts the three arches of the foot. The arches hold the bones of the feet and ankles in their correct position, encourage foot muscles to function efficiently, and act as shock absorbers. Fallen arches are often the cause of tired, aching feet.

To evaluate your ankle and foot alignment, have a friend or your yoga teacher stand behind you and check the relationship of your heels and ankles. If the heels and ankles lean inward or outward, this misalignment affects the feet, knees and hips. Check to see if one foot leans in or out more than the other. Are your arches lifted or flattened?

Fingers and Toes Entwined

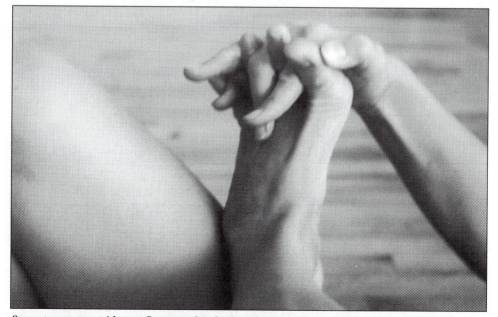

Separate your toes with your fingers and make them free and independent!

By diligently practicing the Fingers and Toes Entwined exercise described on the following page, you can begin to undo a lifetime of damage to your feet. You will be surprised to discover that all 10 toes will come back to life if you commune with them through stretching and massage.

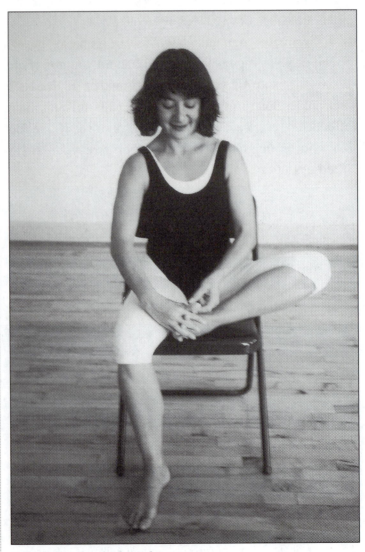

Take off your shoes and stretch your toes.

Fingers and Toes Entwined
While Seated

1. Sit in a chair or on the floor. Bend your left knee and take hold of the left foot with both hands.
2. Interlace the fingers of the right hand with the toes of the left foot, as illustrated. Slide the base of your little finger into the base of the little toe, your next finger into the base of the next toe until all your fingers and toes are firmly connected. Then spread your fingers wide apart.
3. Extend through your heel and stretch the toes toward your left knee. Hold for at least one minute and repeat on the opposite side. When you release your fingers, notice how the color of your feet has improved from increased circulation.

If you can't get the fingers between the toes, try placing the heel of your hand on the ball of the foot and wrapping your fingers over the top of the toes. Press the toes toward the knee and stretch them apart as best you can.

As you become adept at stretching your feet, you can simultaneously press the various reflex points on the big toe with your thumb. (For specific points, check a foot reflexology chart.) Use the thumb on your opposite hand to give the big toe an extra stretch by pulling it even farther away from its neighbor. Stretch the little toe and big toe in opposite directions. Pretend that you are "sawing" your fingers in between your toes. Dig deep into the base of any toe that is especially stiff and stubborn, to show your feet that you really mean business and that you are sorry for abusing them all these years.

Keep the base of the fingers and base of the toes connected long enough so that the space between the toes expands. Increase the length of time daily.

Note position of foot on seat of chair. More flexible people can increase hip flexibility by positioning the foot on top of the thigh.

Fingers and Toes Entwined Lying Down

Lie on your back, a folded blanket or book under your head. Bend both knees and place both feet on the floor close to your bottom. Bring your right knee toward your chest and place the side of your right foot on your left thigh near your knee. Hold the right foot with your left hand. Interlace the fingers of the left hand with the toes of the right foot, connecting the base of your fingers with the base of the toes. Keeping the fingers and toes entwined, extend through your right heel and stretch your toes toward your right knee.

To increase the stretch in your hips while stretching your toes, lift your left foot off the floor and bring your left knee closer to your chest. Your right hand can be used to support the right knee or to keep your right foot from slipping off your left thigh. (If you have trouble reaching your toes, place a big book or bolster under your left foot and add more height under your head.) Release the right leg. Repeat these instructions with your left leg.

The more painful it is to stretch your toes, the more, I assure you, that you need it! Smile, breathe slowly, and let go of the pain and stiffness. Facing the little pains in the feet will help you to avoid the greater pains in your body.

More Ways to Stretch the Toes

Many of my students ask me what I think about using pedicure spacers, cotton balls or other spacers in between the toes. While they may help a little bit, they are not a substitute for stretching and exercising the feet and toes. Most problems with the feet are mechanical. While it is helpful to walk around with toe separators

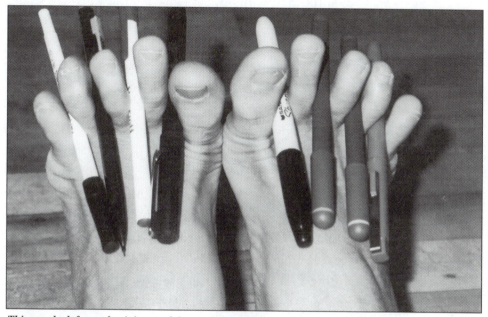

This may look funny, but it is a useful way of expanding the spaces between your toes.

and other orthopedic paraphernalia, nothing takes the place of proper exercise to restore balance to the feet, ankles and rest of the body.

Here is another yoga foot therapy suggestion that has helped many people. In medical classes at the world-renowned Ramamani Iyengar Memorial Yoga Institute in India, teachers insert slender sticks and twigs in between the students' toes. Our Westernized alternative is to replace twigs with pens and pencils of various thicknesses. A practical way to insert them into the base of the toes is to sit on the floor with your feet straight out in front of you, bend the knees to bring the feet within reach, and then experiment with inserting the pens in between the base of each toe. Save the thicker pens for the big toes. If your toes are very tight and painful, start with thinner pens, yet thick enough so that they force you to stretch your toes wider apart. Use your common sense. This usually feels from slightly uncomfortable to painful, but if done sensibly it is stimulating and effective. Keep the pens in between the toes for several minutes. (You can sit with the legs straight, toes stretched toward your face as illustrated.) Gradually increase the length of time.

Yoga places great emphasis on the importance of stretching the feet while stretching the rest of your body. Proper movement and alignment of the feet are often the most effective remedy for foot problems. By paying attention to your feet, spreading the toes and lifting the arches, you will discover that your shoes no longer wear out unevenly, your calluses soften and the spaces between your toes expand as you walk down the road of life.

Foot Reflexology

Many people react with pain when I press certain parts of their feet, a sure sign that their feet need more stimulation. A healing art known as Foot Reflexology teaches that the 72,000 nerve endings on each foot connect to different body areas, and that the toes and their bases contain nerves that extend to glands and sensory organs within the head. Although each toe relates to specific organs within the head, the big toe is said to relate to all glands and organs within the entire head.

Reflexology has its roots in ancient Chinese acupressure and theorizes that by massaging the nerves in the feet, we stimulate corresponding body areas. Ill-fitting shoes place uneven pressure on these nerve endings, whereas walking barefoot, massaging and stretching the feet, improves circulation and benefits the health of the whole body.

According to yoga philosophy, the connection of hands and feet completes the circuits of energy that flow through fingers and soles, and through the right and left sides. In forward-bending postures, the hands often hold the ankles or soles of the feet. By pressing the hands on the ankles or feet, you create resistance and expand the space in joints and spinal vertebrae. This pressure also promotes healthy circulation in the arteries and veins in the bottom of the feet. According to Reflexology, compression massage, even simply placing the hands on the feet, helps the blood on its upward journey to the heart and brain.

According to the Bible and other ancient teachings, the feet are symbols of humility and peace. In many yoga postures the feet are brought above the level of the head (as in upside-down poses), or the head is brought down toward the feet, (as in standing and seated forward bends). In more advanced back-bending postures the feet and head actually meet. If it is true that the head is indeed the seat of the ego, this helps to explain yoga's theory that bringing the head and feet together may help to cultivate more humble, introspective and thoughtful characteristics in our personalities. Yoga also

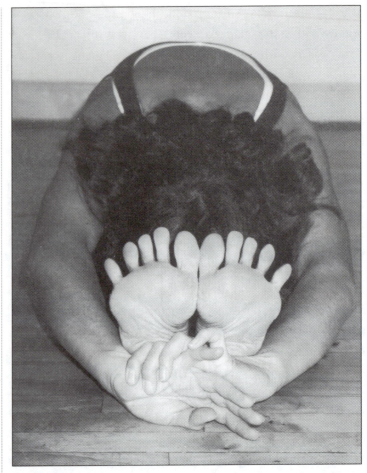

Stretch your toes in all yoga poses. This forward bend stretches the toes and backs of the knees.

emphasizes, however, that before you practice standing on your head or place your body in other unusual positions, you must first "learn to stand on your own two feet."

Your Knees Need Yoga, Too

I can still hear my anatomy instructor rattling on about the knees being the biggest and most complicated joint in the body, while he pointed to the legs of "Miss Bones," the shapely skeleton who dangled faithfully beside his desk.

The knees are between the two longest bones of the body: the femur, or thighbone, and the tibia, or shin bone. The bones of the knee are held together by criss-crossing ligaments, gristle-like structures that join the femur and the tibia to make the knee sturdy and keep it from wobbling. Since almost all the weight of the body passes through the leg bones, thick pads of cartilage called the meniscus act as shock absorbers between the bones when the knee joint is flexed or extended.

These cartilage pads are easily injured. Because of their poor supply of blood, they heal very slowly. Besides torn cartilage, there are at least four other types of knee injuries: sprained ligaments, fractures of the bone joints, wear and tear on the knee cap, (a small, flat triangular bone at the front of the knee) and wear and tear on the muscle tendons.

A quick glance in an anatomy text will help you appreciate the complexities of the knee and show why knees are prone to injury. Exercise that takes the knee joint through its full range of motion is of utmost importance to both prevention of knee problems and repair of injuries.

As in all joints in the body, function is a trade-off between mobility and stability. For example, the shoulder is extremely mobile, but quite unstable and easy to dislocate. The hip is not very mobile, but it is stable. When compared with the hip and shoulder joints for stability, the knee is somewhere in the middle. It is actually one of the most functional joints in the body, allowing us to sit, stand, walk, run, kick, squat and move in hundreds of activities.

As anyone with a knee injury knows, the knees can be mighty unforgiving. When I first began practicing yoga, probably like millions of other Westerners, I strained my right knee attempting to sit cross-legged in the Lotus Pose. When I finally realized that my knee problems were caused by tight hips, I began practicing a series of stretching exercises that gradually gave me enough hip flexibility to sit comfortably on the floor without any complaints from my knees.

Whenever there is a problem in one part of the body, it is always advisable to see how the rest of the body may be causing or contributing to the problem. If the knee joint has been traumatized, it is a good idea to stretch and strengthen the ankle and hip joints, since knee problems are often a reflection of problems at the foot or hip joint. You may remember from the previous section on the feet that if the base of the body is out of balance, strain can occur at the knee. If the hip joints are tight, as they were for me when I first attempted to sit cross-legged, then the rotation needed to sit in this position is forced at the more delicate knee joint instead of coming from the more stable hip joint.

Inflexible joints combined with tight leg muscles force the knees to move in ways inappropriate for their design. Because in our culture the average person chronically tightens muscles, and because we feel this is normal, many people do not realize how restricted their musculoskeletal system is.

The strength and flexibility of the muscles at the front of the thighs (quadriceps), the backs of the legs (hamstrings) and the inner thigh muscles (adductors) all influence the health of the knees. Since most athletic activities involve keeping the knee flexed most of the time, these muscles become tight. Running tightens the hamstrings because the knee is never fully extended and the hamstrings are used as decelerators for the forward-swinging leg, to keep it from moving too far forward. Such repetitive activity tends to tighten both hamstrings and the quadriceps. As the muscles around the knee joint become tighter, they restrict the length of the stride and the freedom of the knee joint. This causes soreness and eventually leads to knee injuries.

A person with an injured knee, or someone with very stiff leg muscles, is generally advised to begin stretching in positions where the knee is kept straight without bearing weight, as illustrated in chapter 3. The knee is most protected when the leg is fully extended. The following leg stretch, described in chapter 3, is recommended for people of all ages, especially those over 50!

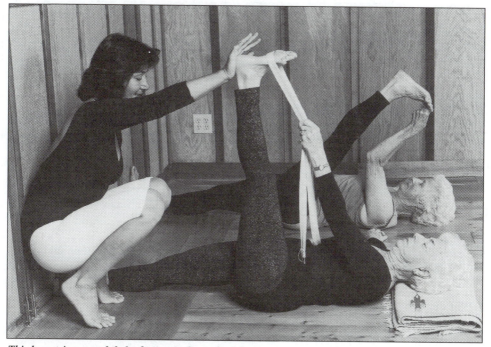

This hamstring stretch helps keep your knees healthy.

Practice the Hero (or Heroine) Pose for Healthy Knees *(Virasana)*

In our chair- and car-oriented culture, most older adults lose the natural ability to sit comfortably between their feet. The Hero Pose is especially difficult for runners and cyclists, who often come to yoga with knee problems and extremely tight front thigh muscles. It is not unusual for new students who have not sat in this position since childhood to first attempt the pose by sitting on a high bolster or stack of blankets, folded lengthwise.

Study the photos below, carefully noting the placement of the blocks and folded sticky mat. If you experience cramping in your feet or pain in your ankles, place

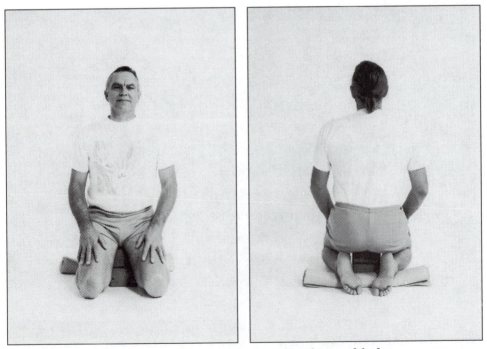

Hero Pose. Note how the props raise the entire torso and cushion the tops of the feet.

a rolled towel, folded blanket or sticky mat under the ankles and feet as illustrated, with the toes on the floor. For stiff feet and ankles, you can also kneel with your knees and shins on two or three neatly folded blankets, with the feet hanging over the edge.

To make the pose more comfortable, it is often helpful to roll a wash cloth, sock or soft rope and place it firmly into the crease behind each bent knee, to increase space in the joints.

How to Practice Hero Pose

1. Begin on your hands and knees with the feet and knees about hip-width apart. Point your toes so that the tops of your feet and ankles are on the floor, toes turned slightly inward. Position your block or bolster behind you in such a way that when you lower your bottom you will end up sitting near the front of the prop.

2. From a kneeling position, slowly lower your bottom to the bolster, blankets, block or floor. If your bottom does not make contact with the floor or prop, or if you experience knee strain, add more height. Place enough support under your bottom so that you can sit upright as illustrated, with your hands pressing down into your thighs.

3. To release, come forward to a kneeling position, with your hands on the floor. Follow Hero Pose with Downward-Facing Dog Pose, described in chapter 4.

If Hero Pose feels impossible no matter how many props you use, try practicing this pose kneeling on a

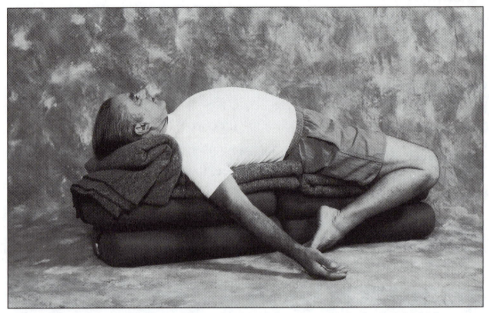

Lying Down Hero Pose is a good way to open the chest and gently stretch the front of the thighs.

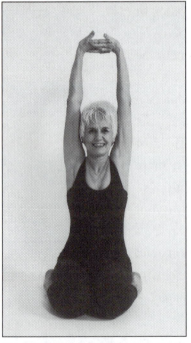

Stretch up both sides of the body evenly in this revitalizing pose.

bed. Place a stack of pillows near the edge of the bed in such a way that you can kneel onto the bed with the pillows between your knees and under your bottom. From a kneeling position on the bed, lower your bottom to the stack of pillows. If your feet feel very stiff, position yourself so that your feet hang off the side of the bed.

The above photo illustrates one of the many ways stiff beginners can practice the Lying Down Hero Pose (*Supta Virasana*). Become comfortable sitting upright in the pose before attempting a lying down variation. The guidance of a teacher is highly recommended.

As you become more comfortable, you can lengthen your spine by stretching your arms upward. Interlock your fingers and note which thumb is in front. Turn the palms out and stretch your arms forward and up. Stretch your trunk up with the arms and draw the arms farther back. Continue stretching upward for several breaths. Release your arms down. Reverse your interlock (opposite thumb in front) and stretch upward again.

Ruth K. Lain at 82:
Yoga Opens Doors to New Friends and interests

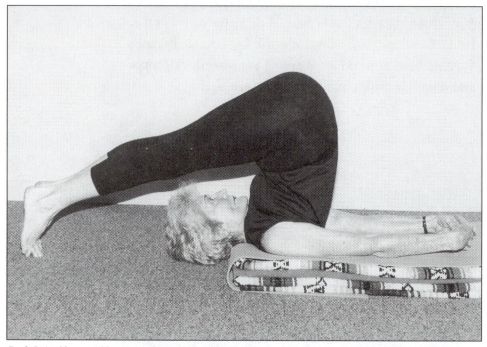

Ruth Lain, 82-year-old yoga teacher, who has practiced yoga since she was 65, demonstrates the Plow Pose.

I feel physically, mentally, emotionally and spiritually better than I ever have in my life. That's an honest fact.

I'm much calmer, and I'm much more stable emotionally and spiritually. Yoga doesn't teach spirituality and meditation, but the support and care of the soul are its by-products.

With yoga, the key word is "aware." Yoga teaches you to be aware of every aspect of your life, including the food you eat. Many people aren't aware of what they do, and yoga helps you with this.

My husband recently died. When anything traumatic happens, yoga is your back-up. When you've been married 52 years, there is such a bond, you cannot just suddenly break that bond. . . . I don't know how I would have survived without yoga. It would have been much harder.

After retiring from public school teaching at the age of 65, I became interested in yoga through Lilias on P.B.S. [Public Broadcasting Service]. At that time my husband and I were living on a farm 40 miles from Corpus Christi, Texas, where there were no yoga instructors—we drove 150 miles to San Antonio. There I had three private lessons before my teacher moved to New York. Totally dedicated to yoga but again without an instructor, I decided to share what I had learned with some of my farm neighbors. Of course, this sharing inspired and challenged me to learn and practice more.

I decided that since I couldn't find a local yoga teacher, I had to become one. Actually, I hauled in unwitting neighbors, relatives and anyone I thought was open enough to try.

My living room class gradually expanded and I started other small classes in abandoned rural schoolhouses and church annexes. After a few years I had six groups in Corpus Christi and was spending a lot of time driving home at night on the highway. My husband and I moved into town and transformed our garage into a studio, called the "Yoga Room," where I now give private lessons and teach nine classes weekly to both men and women of all ages. I also continue with two groups at the Y.W.C.A.

During my lifetime I have had many serious illnesses: 10 operations, a chronic asthmatic condition and a duodenal ulcer. Now because of yoga I feel really good and am never sick. I haven't had asthma since about the first year into doing yoga. I take no medication. Besides physical, mental and emotional health, yoga has opened doors for new friends and interests. I feel truly blessed to be continuously exploring this beautiful way of life.

My personal joy in yoga as well as responsibility to my students encouraged me to study at the Iyengar Institute in San Francisco and to attend workshops with other Iyengar teachers. I've taken week-long and weekend courses with some of the top teachers in the United States. I learned from them, from books and from practicing. There are 8,000 poses in yoga, so there's always something new to learn.

I'm still teaching 10 classes a week and giving five or six private lessons. Recently I had an 80-year-old woman call me and ask, "Am I too old to do yoga?" I asked her, "Can you still breathe? Well then, come for a lesson."

Six

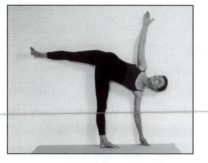

Yoga: A Reliable Companion During Menopause

Actually, aging, after 50, is an exciting period; it is another country. Just as it's exciting and interesting to be an adolescent after having been a child, or a young adult after having been an adolescent. I like it. It's another stage of life after you're finished with this crazy female role.

—Gloria Steinem, interviewed by Cathleen Rountree in *Women Turning Fifty*

Today more women than at any other time in history are approaching or are in the midst of menopause. Within the next 20 years, between 40 and 50 million women in the United States will enter this stage of life.

Menopause itself is changing, in part because the social and economic roles of women have altered so dramatically in the last 50 years, and in part because we understand this transition differently. The work of women like Germaine Greer, Sadja Greenwood, Susan Lark, Christiane Northrup, Gail Sheehy, Susun Weed and many others is redefining this important time in a woman's life. These researchers all recognize the special value of a mind/body discipline such as yoga, especially during menopause. "If you don't already do an hour or more of yoga, t'ai chi, or some other meditative physical activity weekly, begin now," advises Susun Weed in *Menopausal Years, the Wise Woman Way: Alternative Approaches for Women.* And, "It is of the utmost importance for any woman over 45 faced with high-stress professional or personal demands to commit herself to some restorative relaxation measure," echoes Gail Sheehy, in *The Silent Passage: Menopause.*

> Menopause is a time for taking stock, of spiritual as well as physical change, and it would be a pity to be unconscious of it.
>
> —*Germaine Greer,* The Change, Women, Aging and Menopause

What Is Menopause?

Technically speaking, menopause refers to the final menstrual period and the end of a woman's reproductive life. However, most people use the term menopause to mean the year or two of hormonal changes leading up to the cessation of the menses and all of the remaining years of a woman's life.

Menopause, like puberty, is caused by shifts in the balance of hormones within the body. At about midlife, a woman's ovaries, the glands that regulate fertility and the menstrual cycle, reduce their production of estrogen and progesterone. Menstruation becomes irregular and the number of days between periods varies until menstruation finally stops. For most women this occurs in their late 40s or early 50s, although for some this occurs as early as 35.

While these hormonal changes are taking place, some women bleed more frequently than normal or experience dramatically heavier flow. For many women in our culture, changes in their hormonal balance cause uncomfortable "hot flashes" or night sweats. Menopause is associated with a host of other symptoms, including mood swings and depression, urinary problems, vaginal dryness, aching joints, reduced libido and weight gain. Few women experience all of these symptoms, although 75 percent of all menopausal women experience one or two. Some have no major symptoms at all except the end of menstruation.

Menopause also affects women psychologically. Mood swings not unlike those associated with premenstrual tension are reported by some women, while others describe periods of depression, confusion or memory lapses. Many women experience disturbances in their normal sleeping patterns.

However, once the physical changes of menopause are complete, women are free from the powerful hormonal ebb and flow that governed their fertility. They are in a steady state, focused, energized and ready to use the wisdom of their experience. Many women, like Margaret Mead, the famous American anthropologist, feel a new excitement and vitality, which she described as "post-menopausal zest."

While some women sail through menopause virtually symptom-free, others find it distressing. If a woman's identity is tightly bound to being a mother, or if she has not had children, she may grieve the loss of her fertility.

One of the least understood or least tolerated manifestations of the older woman's personality is her withdrawal from the abundantly other-directed behavior patterns of her mothering period, into a more self-directed mode of life, the change more or less coincident with menopause.

—*Barbara Walker,*
The Crone: Woman of Age,
Wisdom and Power

If being sexually attractive is crucial to her feeling valued in her relationships, she may feel the best part of her life is over. Judith Lasater, Ph.D., P.T., in her book, *Relax & Renew: Restful Yoga for Stressful Times*, reminds women that:

Perimenopause [just before menopause] comes at a time when other stressful events are challenging women. Sick or dying parents, career demands, a partner retiring or cutting back on work hours, changing financial status, or children leaving home do little to smooth the effects of the roller-coaster ride of changing hormone levels.

How Culture Affects Our Responses to Menopause

In many cultures menopause is viewed more positively than it is in America, and it is accompanied by fewer negative symptoms. Women may look forward to menstruation's end and the freedom from managing their fertility. In cultures in which old age is honored and women are revered, menopause confers a higher status. In these cultures, menopausal women become the elders who, with their wisdom and experience, guide community life.

As always, our expectations influence outcome. The way we perceive life's stages plays a crucial role in how we experience them. In her excellent book, *Women's Bodies, Women's Wisdom*, Christiane Northrup, M.D., explains how the Celtic cultures view the stages of a woman's life:

. . . the young maiden was seen as the flower; the mother, the fruit; the elder woman, the seed. The seed is the part that contains the knowledge and potential of all the other parts within it. The role of

Though I wrote about living in *The Fountain of Age,* in my personal life I was still being terribly workaholic. So last summer, instead of writing all day I did yoga, I took painting lessons . . . What happens to you after 50, after the reproductive years, more than any other period of your life, depends on what you choose to do. It isn't programmed biologically. To have purpose is essential for vital age.

—Betty Friedan, at age 72

the postmenopausal woman is to go forth and reseed the community with her kernel of truth and wisdom.

In our culture, in spite of many positive changes, aging itself is still hated and feared. In jokes, television shows and greeting cards—all powerful signs of cultural attitudes—we are said to be "finished" or "over the hill" once we reach 50. If we believe that, it's no wonder we perceive menopause as degeneration. However, if we refuse to accept such cultural stereotypes and take charge of the way we think about menopause, it can become the most powerful period in our lives.

Menopause As a Time for Reflection and Re-Direction

Menopause, like other transitional periods in our lives, can be an opportunity to sort out our priorities and celebrate the depth and richness of our experience. If we are at peace with ourselves as mothers or women without children, we may find the freedom from menstruating and managing our fertility liberating. We are at a new stage of our lives. Children, if we have them, are more independent, perhaps even out of the house. Our partners, if we have them, may be experiencing new levels of success or satisfaction. There is time for a different kind of closeness in our relationships. If we live alone, we are more sensitive to our own needs, taking greater pleasure in having things our own way and in the freedom to make our own decisions. We are also more perceptive about ourselves, clearer about our relationships.

Some of us may feel troubled, full of regret for things we've left undone, paths left unexplored. It takes some

When menopause arises as a crisis for us it is sometimes not only the physical symptoms but also the predicament of being a woman undeniably aging in a culture which seems only to value young women.
—*Paddy O'Brien, Yoga for Women*

courage to face that and lay it to rest, so for a time we may suffer. But in general, our perspective is richer and broader. Years of experience have shaped the way we see the world and made us more confident in ourselves.

What Yoga Offers Women During Menopause

At this juncture, the practice of yoga asanas is extremely beneficial, as it calms the nervous system and brings equipoise.

—*Geeta Iyengar,*
Yoga, A Gem for Women

Yoga can be a powerful tool for helping women experience the passage into menopause as a positive event, both physically and spiritually. For women wanting to break free of lifelong negative habits and addictions, practicing yoga provides strength and support. Because it works by balancing the endocrine system, yoga reduces the effects of menopause's hormonal changes. Not only does regular practice of yoga help ease the physical aspects of menopause, but it inspires a spiritual awakening that helps women open to the power and beauty of this profound change.

How Menopause Can Help Us to Expand Our Practice of Yoga

During menopause, many experienced practitioners discover they are more open to exploring the spiritual aspects of yoga. They feel a deep pleasure in the peace and feeling of unity with the universe that they glimpse during their practice. The menopausal years are a time for women to explore and strengthen their spiritual understandings through their open, flowing and intuitive approach to yoga.

Instead of attempting to mold the body into classic postures, many experienced older women teachers advocate experimenting with yoga in a different way—with less focus on control and more on discovery and exploration. There is richness in finding your body's own way into the poses, exploring your strength, fully experiencing the present while consciously releasing the past and making space for the new.

Yoga Postures to Relieve Hot Flashes, Night Sweats and Other Symptoms

For centuries the classic inverted postures such as Headstand and Shoulderstand, as well as various relaxing forward bends and restorative postures, have been valued for their cooling and calming effects. My students tell me these postures are an effective antidote to hot flashes and other common symptoms of menopause. A long stay in Shoulderstand has a particularly quieting effect on the brain and nervous system. According to 96-year-old yoga teacher Indra Devi, Half and Full Shoulderstands are the most important postures for correcting imbalances or hormonal problems in a woman's reproductive system.

Christiane Northrup, M.D., reports that hot flashes, also known as vasomotor flushes, are experienced by 80 to 90 percent of American women during the menopausal years. During hot flashes the surface temperature of the body rises and sweating occurs, sometimes profusely, often around the head and neck. Some women experience hot flashes for only a few months, others for several years. A small percentage report these disturbances for a decade or more.

Scientists are still not sure what causes hot flashes, perhaps the most infamous symptom of the menopausal years. The most widely accepted theory is that these

When I started yoga in 1958 I considered it a tool, the best and most complete tool available, to live physically and psychologically at optimum level. . . . Now that I am 50 years old yoga has once again become a tool for living. I tend to put more stress on enjoyment both in and outside the field of yoga, using the benefits of a balanced yoga practice to enjoy the miracle of life and one's own potential to the fullest possible.

—Dona Holleman, yoga teacher, author of Centering Down

sudden and dramatic increases in surface body temperature occur when your body's thermostat, located in the hypothalamus, is disturbed by hormonal imbalances. Because hot flashes involve the neuroendocrine system, unresolved stress tends to increase them.

Regular yoga practice, as well as other regular exercise such as bicycling or walking, can help alleviate these symptoms. In particular, yoga's inverted poses—such as Handstand, Headstand, Downward-Facing Dog Pose, Shoulderstand, Supported Legs-Up-the-Wall Pose—which position the body completely or halfway upside down, reduce the incidence and intensity of hot flashes and night sweats.

Inverted yoga poses have a measurable effect on what physiologists call hemodynamics—the flow of blood to every organ of the body. They also have a beneficial effect on the glands of the endocrine system that produce the hormones that regulate many of the body's processes. Inverted postures are also cleansing and boost the health of the immune system. According to psychobiologist and yoga teacher Roger Cole, Ph.D., who has conducted extensive scientific studies on the physiological effects of yoga poses:

Turning the body upside down also tricks the body into believing that blood pressure has risen, because the receptors that measure blood pressure are all in the neck and chest region. The body takes immediate steps to lower blood pressure, including a relaxation of blood vessels and a reduction in the hormones that cause retention of water and salt.

On a more subtle level, according to the ancient yogic texts, the inverted postures affect the flow of *prana,* or life-force energy. They draw the prana inward, toward our vital organs, toward the core of the body and away from the surface—the skin. According to some theories, during hot flashes prana is flowing outward from the center, heating the skin.

For experienced students working under the guidance of a teacher, Lying Back Over a Chair and Supported Bridge Pose, also help reduce hot flashes. (See pages 122-123, 137-139 and 214-215.)

Although most women who experience hot flashes seek relief, some researchers believe the increase in the body's surface temperature might serve a useful function. Vickie Noble, in her book, *Shakti Woman,* reminds us that a high body temperature kills bacteria. She and other researchers feel that hot flashes may actually be healthy. When we attempt to shut down the hot-flash process, we might be interfering with a subtle healing mechanism.

Yoga for Easing Mood Swings and Depression

Shifting levels of estrogen and progesterone, both mood-altering hormones, can result in irritability, anxiety and depression during menopause. "In menopause as in puberty, you are going through hormonal changes," says yoga teacher and grandmother Felicity Green. "When a child is going through puberty, we're patient with her. In menopause you have to be patient with yourself. Women should realize this change is normal and natural and give ourselves some time to be quiet."

Herbalist Susun Weed writes in *Menopausal Years, the Wise Woman Way: Alternative Approaches for Women:*

Joint mobility increases rapidly with the focused attention and gentle stretching of yoga postures. Yoga postures, yoga breathing, and quiet, focused meditation tone and soothe the sympathetic nervous system. Regular practice alleviates anxiety. Yoga— not just the postures, but the breathing and focusing exercises as well—helps create strength in the nerves, adrenals, and heart, making sensitivity and irritability an ally rather than a liability.

Forward Bends

In addition to calming the mind and soothing the nervous system, forward bends (see page 133 for

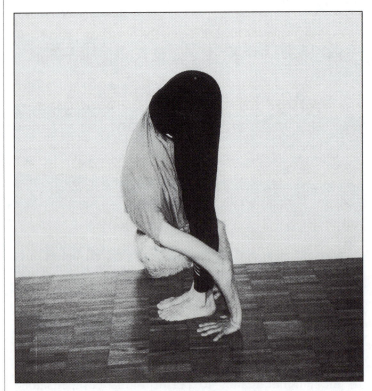

Forward bends calm the mind and soothe the nervous system.

instruction) gently stretch the spine and lengthen the entire back of the body. They encourage an attitude of surrender and acceptance that relieves stress and alleviates many of the negative symptoms associated with menopause.

A simple Standing Forward Bend inverts the upper body and brings the head below the heart. In this position the pituitary gland is stimulated. This small gland in the center of the brain is involved in the regulation of blood sugar levels and body temperature.

Forward bends also gently compress the abdomen, massaging the uterus and other abdominal organs. When you come out of the pose and release the compression, the organs are bathed in freshly oxygenated blood and you feel refreshed, renewed.

Yoga to Balance Hormonal Changes

Yoga helps modulate mood swings and reduce fear and anxiety by helping to balance a woman's changing hormones. Many of the symptoms commonly associated with menopause, such as aches, pains and irritability, are intensified by stress; therefore, practicing yoga's relaxing, restorative poses helps ease them.

While the ovaries decrease their production of androgenic hormones—the hormones associated with sexual response, libido and a general sense of well-being during menopause—other parts of the body, such as the adrenal and pineal glands, actually increase their hormonal output. Unfortunately, in many older women the adrenals are damaged by habitual stress, poor nutrition, environmental pollution or other problems. The failure of the adrenal glands to perform this compensatory function may produce symptoms such as mood swings, fatigue or depression that are commonly attributed to menopause.

Yoga poses, such as twists and backbends, improve the functioning of the adrenals, helping to increase the amount of estrogen in the body. These poses also stimulate the kidneys, promoting healthy elimination of metabolic by-products.

Inverted Poses to Alleviate Fatigue

For me, these last six months, I just crave going upside down. You just crave it. It takes the place of chocolate addiction.

—Judi Flannery-Lukas, yoga teacher at midlife

Fatigue is a signal that the body needs to rest, repair itself, restore its energy. When you are tired, it is not the time to exert yourself with strenuous exercise. This is especially true during menopause. Inverted poses are famous for reducing fatigue, feelings of heaviness or lethargy. They not only improve circulation and increase blood flow to the brain, they calm and soothe the emotions. These poses literally change our perspective. It never ceases to amaze me how different the world looks after a long stay in Headstand and Shoulderstand, or in easier inversions such as Legs-Up-the-Wall Pose. (See chapter 11, Restful Inversions.)

Menstruating women often feel heavy and tired at certain points in their cycle. This fatigue can be attributed, in part, to congestion in the pelvic organs. Inverted poses are especially beneficial to these women in the 10 days prior to, and the days immediately following, their menstrual period. Inverted poses, however, are not recommended during menstruation itself.

When you feel too tired to do anything, practice supported inversions. If you are not yet familiar with Supported Shoulderstand, then scoot close to a wall and put up your legs. If you fall asleep, it will be a deep, refreshing rest. You can even lie with your legs up against a headboard or wall in bed.

If you have a headache as well as fatigue, practice Supported Half-Plow Pose and Supported-Legs-Up-the-Wall Pose. You can also use bolsters to help you rest in

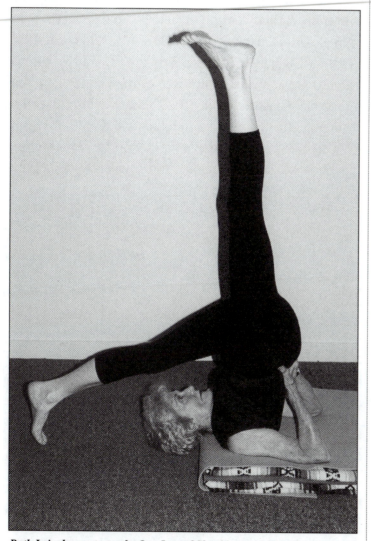

Ruth Lain demonstrates the One-Legged Shoulderstand. This Shoulderstand variation refreshes the legs and strengthens the back.

various positions. Supported Dog Pose and supported forward bends prior to (or after) supported inversions are also healing and restorative.

Poses to Regulate the Menstrual Cycle

A common problem during the perimenopausal years is premenstrual tension resulting from delayed menstrual periods. Upside-Down Bow Pose and Lying Back Over a Chair, where the pelvis opens and the adrenal glands are activated to produce estrogen, may help regulate the menstrual cycle. Backbends are also known to stimulate the ovaries and fallopian tubes.

On the other hand, some women approaching menopause get their periods too frequently, sometimes

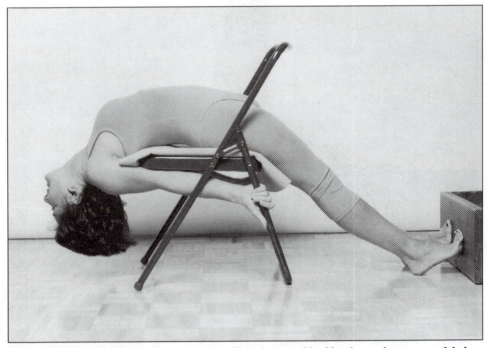

Suza Francina demonstrates Lying Back Over a Chair. Supported backbend poses have a powerful physiological effect. They nourish the nervous system and increase the efficiency of the glandular system.

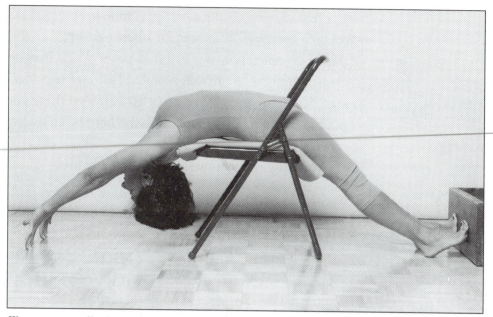

Women cannot afford to neglect these tremendously beneficial backbends. Note how the whole front of the body is stretching.

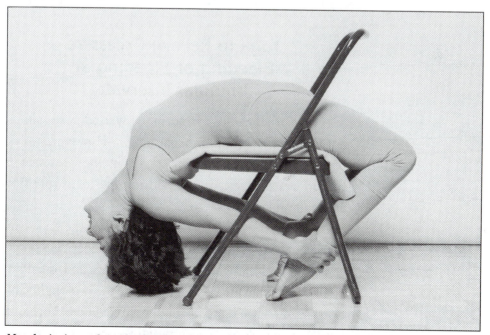

More beginning students should practice as illustrated on page 30. Bolsters may be needed under the head to keep the neck and back comfortable.

as often as two or three times a month. Their cycles become erratic. These women often ask whether they should completely avoid inverted poses while they are menstruating. The answer is individual and requires a high degree of body awareness. To help you determine what is best for you, please seek the help of an experienced teacher.

According to yoga master B.K.S. Iyengar:

> *This "in-between-period bleeding" is not the same as menstrual bleeding. The in-between bleeding may be caused by irritation within the uterus. For example, if after seven days of a regular period the flow has decreased, the yoga practice should be adjusted to further decrease bleeding. Exertion, poses that stimulate the ovaries, may increase the flow and prolong the period.*

Yoga to Relieve Excessive Bleeding or Bleeding at Irregular Intervals

If menstrual cycles are normal, inverted poses should not be practiced during menstruation. However, in case of certain menstrual disorders or in the presence of fibroid cysts, inverted poses during the menstrual flow are recommended.

Inverted poses and backbends stimulate the endocrine glands and correct their function. Any endocrine disorder can also be improved by yoga postures and breathing practices (pranayama), which involve the prolonging and restraining of the breath and help regulate hormonal levels in the blood. These practices should be learned under the guidance of a teacher.

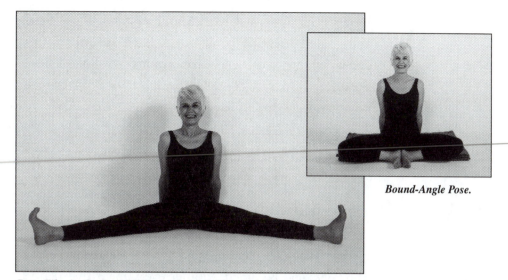

Bound-Angle Pose.

Betty Eiler in the Seated Wide-Angle Pose. The centeredness and symmetry of this pose are very soothing.

To relieve bleeding in between normal periods, it is recommended that women practice healing postures such as Seated Wide-Angle Pose, Seated and Lying Down Supported Bound-Angle Pose and inverted poses.

Yoga to Alleviate Pelvic Congestion

Women often experience a feeling of heaviness and congestion in the first months after their periods have stopped. This is an excellent time to make dietary improvements and to consider a body-cleansing program. Increasing fresh fruits and vegetables will help reduce feelings of heaviness in the abdomen.

All inverted poses, forward bends, the Bound-Angle Pose (both sitting upright with the soles of the feet together and Supported Lying Down Bound-Angle Pose, described on page 134) and Wide-Angle Pose, help reduce pelvic congestion. Headstand,

Lying Back Over a Chair, Shoulderstand, Plow Pose and seated forward bend poses have specific influences on the psycho-neurohormonal system. These postures help reduce tension and thus help reduce menopausal symptoms.

Upside-Down Poses After the Menstrual Period

The classic yoga texts, *Light on Yoga* by B.K.S. Iyengar and *Yoga, a Gem for Women*, by his daughter, Geeta Iyengar, recommend that Headstand and Shoulderstand be practiced after every menstrual period to ensure an inner dryness once the bleeding has stopped. Some experienced teachers caution women against switching too quickly to their usual, more active practice after menstruation. Women who follow the recommended gentle, supported forward bend and restorative practice during the menstrual period and then resume a routine of more strenuous standing, backbending and balancing poses immediately after the period stops may run the risk of overexerting themselves. Some teachers believe that this may contribute to health problems as one gets older, especially during the perimenopausal years.

It seems wise to consider the yoga practice immediately following one's period as a healing practice. Inverted poses and their variations heal the reproductive organs, the organs affected by menopause. Iyengar and other respected teachers recommend a long, quiet stay in Headstand or Shoulderstand, without too many variations. Iyengar writes, "Straight asanas keep you cool, calm, quiet, and when that feeling has come, the mind gets subdued."

The long, motionless holding of inversions opens the door to a state of meditation. It is during and after the peaceful practice of inversions that one experiences poise, peace and stillness at a deeper level. A long stay in the poses quiets and strengthens the nervous system, an invaluable gift at all stages of life, but most especially during the menopausal transition.

According to B.K.S. Iyengar:

> *More than Sirsasana (Headstand), Sarvangasana (Shoulderstand) is helpful because the pituitary gland is not stimulated as much as it is in Sirsasana. That is why the feeling after Sirsasana is very different. . . . That is why I often say that after Sarvangasana the backbends will not be suitable. You do Sirsasana then you do backbending because the pituitary is already active and you can do better back-bendings. But after Sarvangasana you cannot do a backbending course.*

Standing Poses Also Help Relieve Menopausal Symptoms

Standing poses such as Triangle Pose and Half-Moon Pose, with the support of the wall to open the pelvic region, and revolved variations of these poses are also enormously beneficial in helping women adjust to menopause. Standing poses strengthen the whole body, especially the feet and legs; they are tremendously grounding, helping us to re-establish and deepen our connection to the earth. They build confidence and can help us "stand on our own two feet" again. However, if your legs feel heavy and fatigued, listen to your body and take care not to exhaust yourself with long holds in vigorous standing poses. Standing poses practiced against a wall can be helpful when there is dysmenorrhea—pain in the groin, abdomen or pelvis. A moderate standing pose practice such as Triangle and Half-Moon Pose, standing forward bends and Lying Down Big Toe Pose, may help alleviate pain and fatigue in the legs.

When your legs feel heavy and tired, especially during your period, or if your cycle is erratic, it is refreshing to start your practice with supported lying down postures. Lying Down Hero Pose, Lying Down Bound-Angle Pose or simple Lying Down Cross-Legged Pose are all relaxing and restorative.

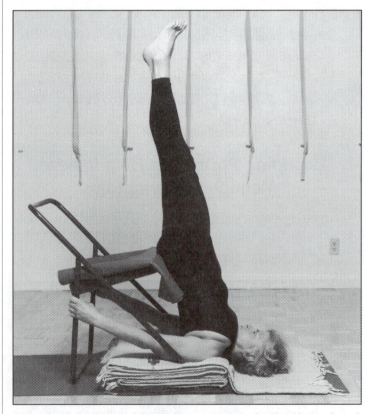

Using the chair allows Malchia Olshan to remain in the Shoulderstand much longer.

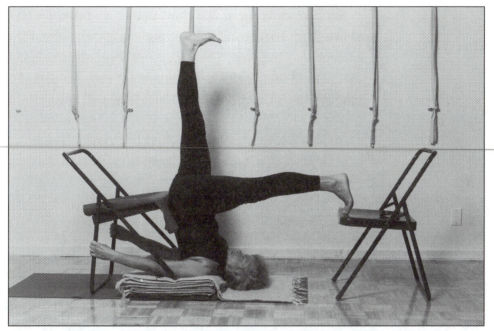

One-Legged Shoulderstand with a Chair helps beginners keep their backs straight.

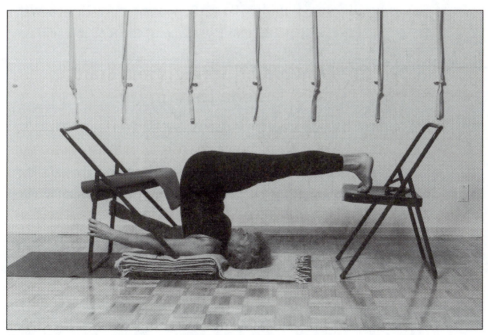

Resting the toes on a chair helps you to straighten and lift your back.

Supported lying down poses followed by Lying Down Big Toe Pose, both straight and with the leg extended to the side, all work to relieve stiffness and tiredness in the legs. When you are not on your period, practice Legs-Up-the-Wall or other inverted poses.

Swollen Legs, Ankles and Varicose Veins

All poses discussed previously, especially inverted poses, are useful for relieving swollen legs and ankles and problems with varicose veins. A long stay (5 to 15 minutes) in simple Legs-Up-the-Wall Pose is highly recommended. Especially if you are standing for long periods of time or involved with sports or athletic activities, as soon as you can conveniently do so, put your feet up on the wall and allow the swelling to decrease. Supported Bridge Pose, Supported Legs-Up-the-Wall Pose, all help decrease swelling of the feet and ankles.

A Word on Stiffness and Starting Yoga Later in Life

People who have not exercised for many years and whose diets are heavy on sugar, caffeine, meat and processed foods commonly experience weight gain and swelling of the joints. A type of stiffness may come into the body that is due not only to lack of movement but also to toxicity. Often these people find it difficult to practice yoga, but they are among those who need it the most.

In these cases, the yoga props described in chapter 3 are especially useful. Without props, people with little energy and many problems often lose heart. Props encourage the body to open and lengthen gradually.

With the help of a wall, people of all ages and conditions can begin practicing the standing poses and simple inversions. Lying back on bolsters and blankets, almost everyone can practice gentle backbends. Forward bends can be practiced sitting on a prop that adds height or with the support of a chair. Again, Supported Lying Down Bound-Angle Pose to open the groin and hips and restore energy is highly recommended.

It is important for women who feel very stiff and rigid prior to and after the time of menopause, to realize that this need not be a permanent condition. If you practice yoga faithfully, the stiffness will leave. With yoga and nutritional support, the body can be cleansed, renewed and rejuvenated. However, without healthy movement, pain and stiffness, especially if masked by medication, can settle deeper, leading to arthritis, osteoporosis and other health problems.

Menopause Practice Guide

The following is a sample sequence of poses to stimulate the ovaries and pituitary gland to produce more hormones. This series has a calming, soothing, quieting effect on the nervous system and, if practiced regularly, helps ease menopausal symptoms. These postures provide a good foundation on which to build a yoga practice that will help maintain a woman's well-being during her menopausal years and beyond.

- Standing Forward Bend with your bottom against a wall (Wall Hang; see page 133)
- Dog Pose (hanging from a strap if available, or with the head supported; see chapter 4, page 73)

- Supported Lying Down Bound-Angle Pose
  (see page 135)
- Supported Legs-Up-the-Wall Pose
  (see chapter 11, page 222)
- Supported Bridge Pose (lying back on bolsters or
  blankets; see pages 138 and 215)
- Supported Child's Pose (see page 140)
- Lying Down Bent-Knee Twist (see page 142)
- Supported Deep Relaxation Pose
  (see chapter 12, page 246)

Experienced students can practice Headstand (either with the head on the floor or practiced between two chairs, as illustrated on page 54) and Shoulderstand, after the Standing Forward Bend and Downward-Facing Dog Pose. More flexible students (those who can bend forward in seated forward bends without strain) can vary their practice with supported seated forward bends before Deep Relaxation Pose.

Standing Supported Forward Bend at the Wall (Wall Hang)

Standing forward bends are halfway upside-down positions that bring the head and neck below the level of the heart. In this variation, known as Wall Hang, you lean your bottom against the wall and bend your torso forward. The whole back of your body releases and lengthens, tension flows out of your body, and the mind quiets down and feels calmer. By remaining with the head hanging down for a half minute or longer, the pituitary gland, located in the center of the brain, is stimulated.

How to Practice
Standing Supported Forward Bend at the Wall

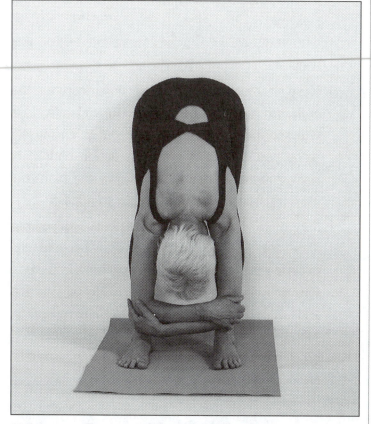

Wall Hang is a relaxing forward bend that brings your head below the level of your heart.

1. Stand tall against a wall with your feet hip-width apart. Keeping your bottom pressing back against the wall, step forward about 12 to 16 inches. The distance from the wall depends on your height and flexibility. Keep your feet hip-width or a little wider apart and breathe out as you release your torso forward.

2. It usually feels relaxing to fold your elbows and allow the weight of your arms and torso to gently stretch your body toward the floor (without bouncing or straining). If tightness in the back of the legs makes this position uncomfortable, practice with your elbows or hands on a chair seat or other support.

3. Keep your legs straight and the quadriceps muscles at the front of the thighs pulled up and active. You will see the definition of the front thigh muscles when you contract them. This action both stabilizes your knee joints and allows the hamstring muscles at the back of the thighs to release.

4. Stay in this Supported Standing Forward Bend for about one-half to one minute. As you become more experienced, you will enjoy remaining in the pose longer. To come up, place your hands on your legs and inhale deeply as you return to standing upright. Step back to the wall and stand tall with your back relaxed against the wall. Feel the calming, soothing effect of this pose.

Supported Lying Down Bound-Angle Pose

Lying Down Bound-Angle Pose can be practiced by simply lying flat on the floor, with the soles of the feet together. However, practicing this position with support from bolsters and blankets opens the chest, abdomen and pelvis and allows the body to relax deeply. Extra support under the forearms, knees and outer thighs makes the pose supremely comfortable. This pose is

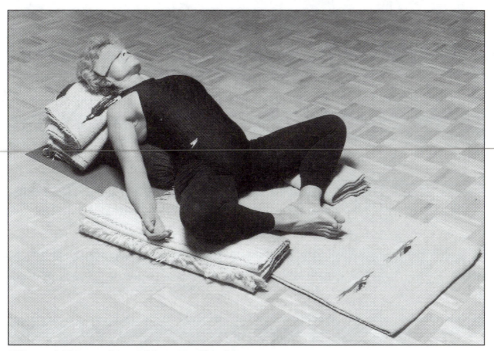

This nourishing pose is one of the great gifts of yoga.

beneficial to those with high blood pressure, headaches and breathing problems. It is a key pose to practice during the menstrual period and menopause transition. It relieves tension and constriction in the abdomen, uterus and vagina and may help balance hormonal processes. The centering, balancing effect of this pose helps reduce mood swings and depression.

How to Practice Supported Lying Down Bound-Angle Pose

As in other supported poses, the height of the support under your back depends on your height and flexibility. New students can start with less height or with one or two blankets folded lengthwise.

1. Sit in front of the bolster or blankets. The edge of the support behind you should touch your tail-bone. Place a double-folded blanket (or two single-folded blankets) at the far end of the bolster to support your head when you lie back. Sit for a few breaths with the soles of your feet together, your fingers on the floor slightly behind your bottom.

2. Use your arms for support as you lower your back and head onto the bolster or blanket. Tuck the double-folded blanket under your neck and head so that your forehead is slightly higher than your chin. Your head should feel comfortable, neither too high or too low. Be sure the bolster supports you from your sacrum to the top of your head. If you feel discomfort in your back, try repositioning your back on the bolster—you may be too high or too low on the bolster. If you still feel strain, decrease the height under your back.

3. Bring the soles of your feet close to your body. Place a long rolled blanket under your outer thighs. The height of these blankets should adequately support the weight of your legs so that your back and knees relax. Your knees should be level. If one knee is much higher, place extra support under the lower knee. Many people also feel more relaxed with the support of a folded blanket under their forearms. Blankets can be folded lengthwise and carefully positioned to support both the legs and arms.

4. When you feel comfortable, remain still in the pose for as long as you like, 10 to 20 minutes or longer. Observe the quiet flow of your breath. To come out of the pose support your thighs with your hands.

Before sitting up, straighten your legs, allowing them to fall evenly away from the midline. Some people prefer lying flat before sitting up. You can turn to your side with your knees bent, move the bolster out of the way, and lie flat on the floor before sitting up, if you prefer. When you feel ready, bend your knees, turn to your side and slowly sit up.

Supported Bridge Pose

Supported Bridge Pose is a combination gentle supported backbend and mild inverted position. You can clearly see and feel the opening of the chest and heart area as you place your body in this pose. It is restful for the heart and may help balance blood pressure and hormonal secretions. It has a calming effect on the mind and nervous system and helps prevent and relieve headaches. Placing your head lower then the rest of your body with the chest open is soothing, refreshing and removes lethargy and depression. It also helps drain fluid from the legs after long periods of standing.

How to Practice Supported Bridge Pose

1. Study the photo on the next page and note how the support under the back and legs is placed end-to-end to accommodate the length of the body. The height of the support depends on the length of your torso and the flexibility of your back. New students can begin with one or two single-folded blankets and gradually increase the height. Six to 12 inches in height works well for most people. Taller people

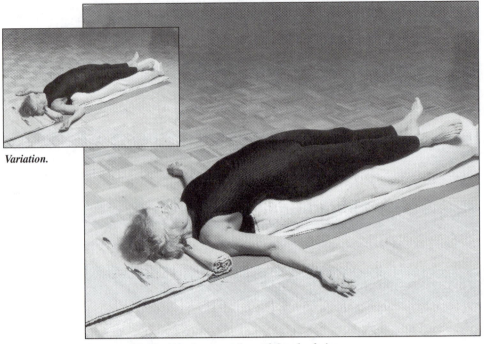

Variation.

Supported Bridge Pose is extremely restful and calming.

can add height to bolsters by placing one or more blankets on top of the bolsters. Make sure that your support is level. You can also place a block under your heels. If your support tends to slope down at the base, add support under your heels.

2. Sit down on the folded blankets or bolsters, either with your legs straight out in front of you or straddling the support. Position yourself near the end of the support so that when you lie down your head is near the far end. Use the support of your arms as you lie down. Slowly slide off the end until the back of your head and shoulders rest flat on the floor.

3. Notice how you feel. If you had difficulty lowering your shoulders to the floor, your support may be too

high. If your lower back feels strain, bend your knees and place your feet either on top of the support or on the floor on either side. Relax your throat and chin. Lengthen and release your neck. If your neck feels jammed, experiment with a small rolled towel at the base of your neck, or roll one end of a folded blanket and tuck it under your neck, with the rest of the blanket under your head as illustrated.

4. When you feel comfortable, close your eyes and cover them. Relax your arms out to the side at a comfortable angle, or with your elbows bent, arms relaxing back just above your shoulders ("baby arms").

Stay in Supported Bridge Pose as long as you feel comfortable, up to 10 or 15 minutes. When you feel ready to come out, remove the eye cover and slowly slide in the direction of your head, until your whole back and bottom are on the floor. Relax for a few more breaths with your lower legs supported by the height. Then bend your knees, turn to your side and slowly sit up.

Bolsters are highly recommended both for their height and convenience. Students consistently report that they practice supported poses much more regularly at home after purchasing bolsters. Consider them an investment in your health for years to come! (See chapter 10 for more benefits of supported backbends.)

Child's Pose

Child's Pose is the natural pose babies and young children assume for rest and relaxation. Interestingly, with the arms extended it is also a universal gesture of worship. This pose not only relieves tension in the back

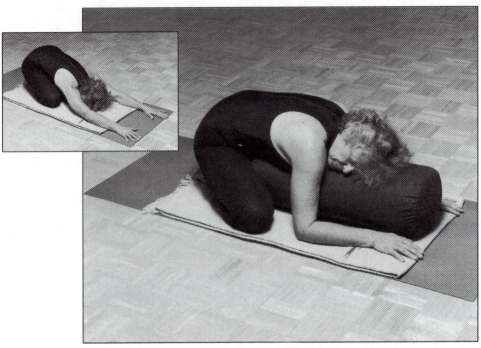

Child's Pose is soothing and relieves tension in the back.

but gives a feeling of comfort and security. Without props it can be practiced between repetitions of active weight-bearing poses like Downward- and Upward-Facing Dog Pose or Right-Angle Handstand. It effectively relieves the lower back ache that comes from standing or sitting still too long. During times when life feels overwhelming and all you want to do is crawl back into bed and hide, try retreating for a few minutes in Child's Pose. With the body supported on a bolster or blankets, it feels like you're giving yourself a warm hug.

How to Practice Child's Pose

1. Kneel on a padded surface such as a carpet, yoga mat or folded blanket with your feet and knees

about hip-width apart, and your bolster or stack of folded blankets placed lengthwise in front of you.

2. Fold more padding under your knees and shins if needed. (See Hero Pose, chapter 5.) Point your toes directly backwards, keeping your feet in line with your calves. Slowly lower your bottom toward your heels. If you experience strain in your knees, place a small towel, folded lengthwise, deep into the crease at the back of your knee to create more space in the knee joints. For discomfort in your ankles or tops of the feet, place a folded towel or sticky mat under the front of the ankles and let the feet hang over the roll, as illustrated in Hero Pose, chapter 5.

3. Separate your knees wide enough to place the bolster or blankets between your thighs as illustrated. To deeply relax and let go in Child's Pose, your torso should be supported by the bolster and your thighs. Your chest should relax on the bolster. Add more blankets if needed. Allow your bottom to move back toward your heels. Many people find Child's Pose easier than Hero Pose, as it can be practiced even if your bottom doesn't touch your heels.

4. If you feel uncomfortable or have trouble breathing, try moving the support in front of you farther away. Some people are more comfortable with their belly off the bolster.

5. Turn your head to the side as illustrated. Relax your chin. If you feel uncomfortable with your head to the side, rest on your forehead with your chin tucked toward your chest. Breathing should feel easy and relaxed. You can hug the bolster or let the arms be passive, as illustrated. Relax in this

position about three minutes. Turn your head to the opposite side when you are halfway through holding the pose. To come out of the pose, place your palms on the floor, under your shoulders. Inhale and sit up slowly on your heels. If your bottom doesn't touch your heels, simply stay in a kneeling position. Then bring one leg forward, placing your foot on the floor. Press your hands on the forward thigh and come back to a standing position. (Refer to chapter 13 on how to use a chair if you have difficulty coming up off the floor.)

People with very stiff knees or ankles may find they need to practice on a thick stack of blankets, either with the toes hanging off or with an extra blanket placed lengthwise under the shins. As in other poses, most problems can be overcome with the help of a teacher or by experimenting with the thickness and placement of the folded blankets and towels.

For people whose feet and knees do not feel comfortable on the floor even with support, or who cannot get up and down from the floor without assistance, practice kneeling and relaxing forward in bed, with pillows or blankets under your bottom and torso, feet hanging off the bed, as described in chapter 5 for Hero Pose.

Lying Down Bent-Knee Twist

I always remind my students, "If you do nothing else, do some gentle twists to relax your neck and back before you go to bed." Gentle floor twists help prevent and relieve lower back pain caused by muscle tension. They also reduce cramps and indigestion and tone the abdominal area.

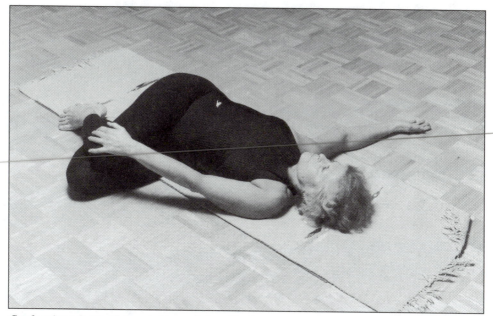

Gentle twists take the kinks out of your neck and back.

How to Practice Lying Down Bent-Knee Twist

1. Lie down with your knees bent, feet flat on the floor, your upper and lower body in line. If your head tilts back, place a folded blanket under your head. Bring your arms in line with your shoulders, palms up, hands actively stretching away from each other to open your chest. Allow your back to relax toward the floor.

2. Still keeping your feet flat, lift your hips up off the floor to move them gently to the left. Lower your hips back down. Bend your knees toward your chest, and slowly lower your knees to the right.

3. Stretch your left arm away from your knees. Your right arm can stay in line with your shoulders, or you can increase the stretch by placing your right hand

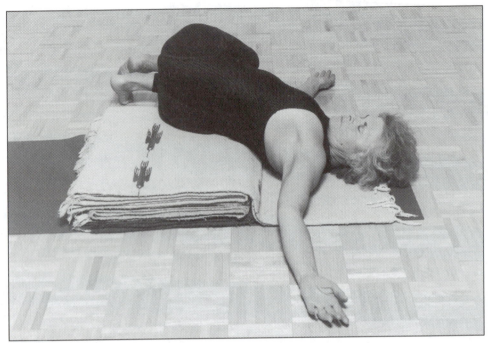

Lying Down Bent-Knee Twist with support feels wonderful after Shoulderstand.

on your knees, gently pressing them down. Stay for a few breaths, allowing your body to release into the pose. When you feel ready, on an exhalation use your abdominal muscles to bring your knees back to the center. Move your hips to the right before slowly lowering your bent knees to the left.

If you feel unusual back or shoulder strain, or if your knees do not touch the floor, place a folded blanket under your knees.

More flexible students can practice this, for example, after Shoulderstand, as illustrated above, with a blanket supporting their pelvis and mid-back.

As you become familiar with the postures in this menopause chapter, please bear in mind that a yoga program for women's health problems may include other poses and variations, which are best learned under the guidance of a yoga teacher. Your instructor may give you specific, individualized instructions to follow. Be aware that there are subtle adjustments and refinements that are beyond the scope of a book. I strongly encourage you to seek and work with a knowledgeable teacher who can help you to make yoga a supportive companion during menopause and for the rest of your life.

Yoga Breathing Practices and Menopause

Pranayama refers to breathing practices that involve the prolongation and restraint of the breath. These practices should be learned under the guidance of a teacher. Pranayama plays a vital role in keeping the body healthy, especially during the later years. Such breathwork eases pressures, breaks up congestion and heals by supplying fresh energy to the pelvic region and the organs of the body, and by stimulating and soothing those areas to bring them back to a normal state.

Pranayama helps relieve menopausal problems by stimulating the autonomic nervous system. For those who wish to explore this subject further, B.K.S. Iyengar in his book, *Light on Pranayama,* explains how these breathing practices directly affect our health by stimulating all the *chakras* where energy is stored. Pranayama releases and distributes the energy of the nervous system. It improves the performance of the respiratory, circulatory, nervous and endocrine systems, alleviating problems associated with menopause. Women at midlife and older are especially encouraged to study and begin the practice of pranayama.

Urinary Problems

At menopause, some women experience urinary problems due to weakness of the pelvic floor which tends to become prolapsed. To counter these difficulties, yoga teachers recommend the practice of a technique called *Aswini Mudra.* Aswini Mudra is similar to the Kegel exercise recommended for pregnant women, in which the sphincters are held and released repeatedly. Regular practice of Aswini Mudra tones the perineal area and pelvic floor and increases blood flow to the pelvic region, encouraging the maintenance of healthy vaginal and urethral tissue.

To practice Aswini Mudra, sit in a comfortable position, preferably on a height to help keep your posture open, your spine lengthening. Gently contract the sphincter and vaginal muscles as if trying to hold back urination. The perineum should be held firm and the pelvic floor should feel as if it is being lifted up. Hold the contraction for a few breaths, then release it for a few breaths. Repeat five to 10 times at first, increasing the repetition and duration as you become more comfortable with the practice. Aswini Mudra can be practiced during daily activities while sitting or standing and during many yoga poses.

A five-step program for bladder control is outlined in the book *Staying Dry: A Practical Guide to Bladder Control* by Kathryn Burgio, Ph.D., Lynette Pearce, R.N., C.R.N.P., and Angelo Lucco, M.D., published by the Johns Hopkins University Press. An estimated one in 10 adults—more than 10 million men and women of all ages—suffer from the annoying problem of urinary incontinence. *Staying Dry* dispels the myths and taboos about incontinence, educates readers about the different types of incontinence and the various treatments available, and teaches a series of exercises and strategies that can significantly improve or cure most types of incontinence in a matter of weeks.

EDITOR'S NOTE: *People who have experienced this medical condition can also obtain a basic packet of information by sending a business size self-addressed stamped envelope and $2.00 to: National Association for Continence (NAFC), P.O. Box 8310, Spartanburg, SC 29305-8310.*

Malchia Olshan:
Hot Flashes Become Cool Breezes
in Forward Bends

At age 65, my student Malchia Olshan is a world champion swimmer. She says that practicing yoga has helped her achieve better times at swimming meets now than when she was in high school. Currently, she is the world's third-ranked miler in the masters division. She competes regularly in the United States and abroad.

One morning soon after I turned 50, I looked in the mirror and saw that my skin seemed to have dropped overnight. My waist was hip-size and my arms and legs were filled with gravity creases.

"Aha! Get thee to serious yoga classes," my conscience told me.

Handstands, Headstands and Shoulderstands counteract the dropping waist. Stretching keeps the limbs loose and scares away those gravity creases. Hot flashes become cool breezes in Forward Bends.

I am a competitive master swimmer. My secret to swimming is yoga, yoga and more yoga. Restorative yoga calms the body and brain after hard swim workouts. Before my swims, I'm on the deck doing Downward-Facing Dog.

Yoga makes me feel like a kid. The added bonus is that my grandson Martin was so impressed with my Handstand that he invited me to his kindergarten class for Show and Tell so his friends could see Grandma stand on her head!

Felicity Green:
Yoga is Healing and Strengthening
on Every Level

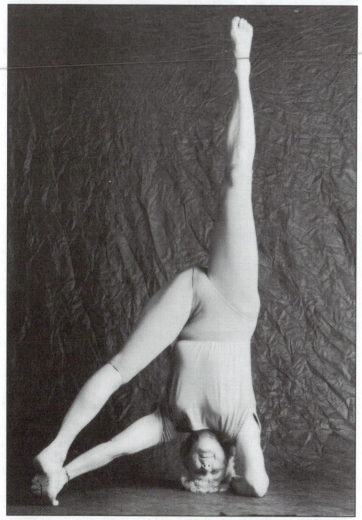

Felicity Green, in her 60s, balances in Headstand with one leg stretching up, the other reaching down.

Felicity Green began practicing yoga after experiencing a traumatic injury to her left shoulder. She had been told by her physicians that her arm and shoulder would never function normally again. Now, 26 years later, she is able to rotate her arm back and forth behind her head and demonstrate a Handstand, Headstand, backbends and other yoga postures that have helped her to develop strength, flexibility and restore full range of motion to her shoulder.

Had Felicity waited 10 or 20 years to begin a yoga and therapeutic exercise program, she would have suffered a functional disability to her left shoulder. The usual consequence of a soft tissue injury is that the body produces pain, inflammation and fibrous tissue in its attempt to heal. However, improvement can still be made even if a person begins yoga many years after an injury, as Felicity confirms:

Hatha yoga is an efficient system that gives you the benefits of cleansing and purifying the body, as well as strength and flexibility. You will gain the feeling of greater freedom and awareness, but as with anything, it's not what you do but how you do it that's important. Asanas must be practiced with a mature awareness to be constructive.

I started yoga as many people do—for a physical reason. But the more important result has been greater emotional stability. Yoga has been healing and strengthening on every level, and I teach to try to help others to discover this for themselves.

I firmly believe that as human beings, we exist on many levels that are intertwined but unfortunately not integrated. The body is the most tangible level and is therefore the most honest feedback system. We carry memories and resistances in our bodies as much as in our minds and psyches. If we pay close attention to the information we gain from the body—for example, our reaction to challenge—and apply that to other aspects of ourselves, the changes become profound.

My own experience and my observations of students over the years have proved that Mr. Iyengar's approach brings about deep and gradual change, not merely an intellectual "flash in the pan." In this, I think, lies the importance of his work for the West, where intellect is given far too much importance.

My aim and direction through yoga is to learn to cooperate with change in a sensitive, refined manner and thereby create peace and harmony.

Seven

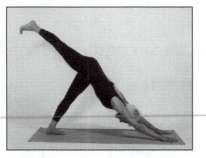

Weight-Bearing Yoga Postures Help Prevent Osteoporosis

Exercise literally can save your life; without it, your body deteriorates. There is no question that if you are inactive your bones will decalcify, leading to osteoporosis, the potentially fatal disease that is so prevalent among older women. Taking time out of your day to attend an exercise class, to take a walk is not frivolous, it's essential.

—LINDA OJEDA, *MENOPAUSE WITHOUT MEDICINE*

The skeleton provides the fundamental structure of the human body. Bones enable us to stand upright and allow us to move when the muscles attached to them are contracted. Bones also protect vital organs. The dense bones of the skull enclose the brain; the slender ribs protect the heart and lungs at the same time as they allow the chest to expand and contract.

How Exercise Strengthens Bones

Our bones are composed chiefly of calcium. They begin developing well before we are born, but are not completed until we are about 25 years old. The reconstruction of bones goes on throughout our lives, in part because bones supply calcium to the rest of the body. Calcium is used by the nerves and in many vital functions. The pattern in which bone rebuilds varies in response to mechanical stress and an individual's activity level.

Bones grow stronger in response to use. In the presence of adequate supplies of calcium in the diet, bone growth is stimulated by any activity in which bones bear weight or muscles pull on them. During these activities, muscles transmit mechanical and bioelectrical signals to bones that cause them to thicken.

If we remain physically active, bones continue a healthy process of regeneration and remain strong. New bone growth, however, is rapidly absorbed if we become immobilized or sedentary. Even athletic and very fit astronauts, living in the weightless environment of space, quickly lose bone mass because their muscles and bones work far less in the absence of gravity.

Osteoporosis is the major cause of bone fractures in older people in general and postmenopausal women in particular. The word "osteoporosis" means "porous bone." As the actual mass of bones decreases, the bones become more susceptible to fractures. In severe osteoporosis, the internal structure of the bones erodes to such an extent that even a slight trauma can cause them to break. Although osteoporosis may affect any bone in the body, the most common sites of osteoporosis-related fractures are the spine (including the neck), wrist and hip.

Fractures of the vertebrae, or bones in the spinal column, occur most often in women within 20 years after menopause and in elderly men. Even tiny fractures in these bones are also the source of the rounded back and loss of height frequently associated with aging. When the bones of the vertebrae are weakened, an ordinary action like bending forward to make a bed or lift a child can be enough to cause a spinal compression fracture. When a fracture occurs, pain may be sudden and severe or chronic and nagging. As additional microfractures develop, the vertebrae collapse into wedge shapes, the upper spine curves forward and height diminishes.

In older osteoporotic men and women, hip fractures frequently occur in the upper portion of the femur or thighbone. Although most of these fractures are surgically repaired, one out of five elderly people with hip fractures dies within a year from complications. Few who recover ever regain complete mobility.

People with osteoporosis are also prone to breaking the bones in the forearm near the wrist. Often, these breaks occur during attempts to stop a fall. Unfortunately, elderly people are prone to falling because of failing eyesight, inner ear disturbances, weak and inflexible muscles, arthritis, slow reflexes, or various neurological conditions.

Osteoporosis and Menopause

Osteoporosis is actually two separate diseases. In one form, osteoporosis develops gradually with age in both men and women. In the other, osteoporosis appears rapidly in women after menopause or after surgical removal of the ovaries. In the second type of osteoporosis, reduced levels of estrogen accelerate bone loss for several years after menstruation ends. Because we are living longer now, we see a great deal more of both types of osteoporosis.

Osteoporosis affects about half the women in the United States over age 45 and 90 percent of those over 75. Although diminishing estrogen levels undoubtedly speed up the loss of bone mass immediately after menstruation ends, recent studies indicate that estrogen deficiency is not the primary cause of hip fractures linked to osteoporosis. The most crucial factor is a sedentary lifestyle. This and other new evidence indicates how important it is for women to remain active and physically fit as they grow older.

Contrary to most people's assumptions about this disease, osteoporosis often appears before menopause. A study of 7,278 hospital discharges following hip fractures shows that the rate for this type of injury for Caucasian women climbs steeply between ages 40 and 44—nearly 10 years earlier than menopause for most women. The hip fracture rate does not increase between the ages 48 to 51 or later, which are usually the menopausal years. Research indicates that bone density actually begins to decrease long before this stage in life sometimes as early as 25 years of age. It is therefore imperative that women take care of themselves well before menopause.

During the climacteric, a woman can experience up to 5 percent loss in bone mass, regardless of how much extra calcium she is taking. After that, the rate of loss

Climacteric refers to the years just before and just after menopause. For most women, the climacteric spans from the early- to mid-40s to late 50s or early 60s, including the pre-menopausal climax years and the post-menopausal years. This entire period constitutes the menopausal years, commonly known as the change of life.

diminishes and levels out as the body adjusts to lower hormonal levels.

A Healthy Lifestyle Reduces Your Risk of Osteoporosis

Because the risk of osteoporosis is increased by a diet high in salt, protein, caffeine and sugar and by the use of alcohol and tobacco, many holistic practitioners maintain that osteoporosis is simply the result of an unhealthy lifestyle that manifests itself about age 50. The typical American diet promotes calcium loss. The amount of sodium in popular snacks, the sodium and phosphorous in processed foods and the phosphorous in red meat and cola drinks all cause calcium to be leached from our bones and excreted in the urine. High-protein, meat-containing diets may also help to deplete calcium. As little as two drinks per day of alcohol, which is a direct chemical poison to the bone-forming cells, may double a woman's risk for osteoporosis. Smoking may also double the risk.

Stress, too, contributes to osteoporosis. When we are under stress, our blood becomes slightly more acidic, which, over time, removes calcium from bones. When we are more relaxed, our blood becomes more alkaline and the bones retain more calcium. Therefore, regular deep relaxation will enhance any program to prevent osteoporosis.

Because bone is restructured constantly, we need calcium and other minerals every day. To supply adequate nutrition, consider adopting a balanced vegetarian diet, recommended for people at risk of osteoporosis. A nutritionist or holistic health professional can help you determine your individual needs. If you tend not to eat sufficient amounts of bone-healthy foods, you may also want to consider taking a complex mineral supplement. Remember, too, that vitamin D helps the body absorb calcium. Just 15 minutes of sunlight a day on your hands and face will stimulate your body to produce all the vitamin D you need.

Inactivity Leads to Bone Loss

Our bodies are meant to be used. In fact, we now know that prolonged rest is disastrous for the muscular and skeletal systems. A hospital patient confined to a bed for a few weeks will suffer as much wasting in the muscles and bones as someone who has aged a decade.

Deepak Chopra, the world-famous expert on mind/body medicine, recommends walking and yoga as the ideal combination of exercises for strengthening and balancing the body. While walking is an excellent, pleasurable exercise and is practical for most people, it only strengthens the bones in the feet, legs, pelvis and, to a lesser extent, the spine. Exercises that strengthen the muscles of the back, such as weight-lifting, help increase the density of the bones in the vertebra. Swimming, though it stimulates bone growth in the forearms and feet, does not strengthen the vertebral bones. In contrast, yoga strengthens bones throughout the body.

A 30-second stay in Downward-Facing Dog or Full Arm Balance (see chapter 4) is usually long enough to convince even the most skeptical athlete that yoga is, indeed, a legitimate weight-bearing exercise, especially strengthening for the wrists and upper body. Attending even one class will demonstrate yoga's superior ability

Aerobics for your heart or weight-training for your muscles may achieve some limited good, but these are not comprehensive enough. . . . The ideal is to balance the whole system, mind and body. It is also vital that exercise give more energy than it takes, a consideration many people tend to ignore. What is needed is a new approach to exercise in which the aim is not to sweat and strain or to pound muscles into shape. . . . The body is not just a shell or a walking life-support system. It is your self intimately clothed in matter. Getting back in touch with this intimacy is very reassuring and delightful, particularly for people who have given up on exercise and become virtual strangers to their bodies.

—Deepak Chopra, M.D.,
Perfect Health: The
Complete Mind/Body Guide

over other form of exercise to remove years of stiffness from the spine, hips and rest of the body.

Look for Exercise Opportunities in Daily Life

To complement your yoga practice, remember to walk in the fresh air in natural light as often possible. Look for exercise opportunities in your daily routines. Get in the habit of walking and riding your bicycle for transportation as well as recreation. Studies show that in spite of all the weight-loss programs, a greater percentage of the American population is overweight than ever before. I firmly believe that this would naturally change if we left our cars at home more and used our legs for daily transportation. Whenever practical, do errands on foot instead of in your car. This can increase the joy of everyday life and help both you and your community to be healthier.

While most of us must make a conscious effort to get enough exercise, people who exercise too much also increase their risk of osteoporosis. For example, female athletes who train excessively or who suffer eating disorders often stop menstruating and become osteoporotic. Premature loss of menstruation is a sure sign that young bones are at risk.

Yoga Helps Prevent Falls by Improving Balance

Yoga not only strengthens bones, it actually helps to prevent falls in the first place by improving balance and coordination, posture and body mechanics. If an older

For me, a long five- or six-mile walk helps. It is at these times that I seem to get recharged. If I do not walk one day, I seem to have on the next day what Van Gogh calls "the meagerness or what is called depression." For a long time I thought dullness was just due to the asphyxiation of an indoor sedentary life. But I have come to learn otherwise. For when I walk grimly and calisthenically, just to get exercise and get it over with, I find I have not been recharged. But if I walk in a carefree way, without straining to get to my destination, my neck and jaw are loose and I look at the sky or the lake or the trees or wherever I want to look, then I am living in the present. And it is only then that the creative power flourishes.

—Brenda Ueland, a writer who set an international swimming record for over-80-year-olds and lived an active and vital life until her death at the age of 93.

person should accidentally stumble and fall, yoga reduces the degree of trauma and likelihood of fractures by strengthening the muscles and making the body more flexible. Strong muscles are better able to control and absorb the impact of falls. Moreover, older people who practice yoga feel stronger, more agile and confident and can get up from falls far more easily than those who are frail and afraid.

Over the years, I have known several students who came to yoga with severe balance problems and needed to use canes. Naturally, these people did not feel secure in the middle of the room. However, they could begin to practice standing poses against a wall, with or without wall ropes. Or they could practice at home, holding onto a built-in counter or sturdy table, as described in chapter 3. It is especially important that students with balance problems not be relegated to practicing yoga in chairs because without weight-bearing exercise, these are the very people who are most often headed for wheelchairs.

Yoga Helps Prevent Height Loss

According to Dr. Christiane Northrup in *Women's Bodies, Women's Wisdom,* decreased height is not always the result of bone loss. Years of poor posture, lack of stretching, or feeling weighed down by life's burdens can also make elderly people shorter than they once were. Some height loss results from the shrinking of spaces between vertebral discs, even when bone density is good. Dr. Northrup observed the least height loss in her patients who regularly practiced yoga. I believe this is because yoga helps to keep the discs between the vertebrae plump and supple and the spaces between them open. Many of my older students report that after practicing yoga for a while, they regain their youthful height.

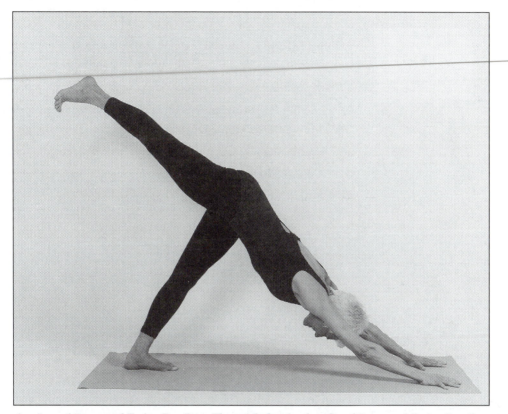

One-Legged Downward-Facing Dog Pose. The weight-bearing benefits of Downward-Facing Dog Pose are intensified by shifting the weight from four limbs to three.

Yoga for Preventing and Counteracting Osteoporosis

The best yoga program for preventing osteoporosis is a balanced practice of asanas (postures), including standing, inverted, seated and lying-down postures. Such a practice stimulates bones to remain strong and healthy as well as improves self-image, coordination and posture. Yoga effectively reeducates the body, cor-recting posture by elongating the spine and stretching and opening the chest.

If you already have osteoporosis, you can practice yoga safely by using props and taking special care to maintain proper alignment. Use extra caution practicing movements such as forward bends that put pressure on already weakened vertebrae. If you are new to yoga, avoid weight-bearing on the spine in poses such as Shoulderstand or Headstand until vertebral fractures heal and your bones have regained more normal strength. As I do for other physical conditions, I highly recommend you seek and work with a qualified yoga instructor.

Betsy Goodspeed:
Yoga Is As Important to Me As Music

I've played the harp professionally for over 30 years. Around the age of 57, I stopped because it just wasn't worth the pain. I had a chronic stiff neck, my right leg was longer than my left, the left hip joint was shot to pieces, the left shoulder was practically frozen, the upper right arm was swollen, and I was so stiff and sore that I had to pull myself out of bed every morning by sheer will power.

Besides playing the harp, I also play the piano, sing, write music and spend long hours at the computer writing. These life-giving creative endeavors took a heavy toll, resulting in punishing pain, endangering my health, perhaps even shortening my life. I paid this stiff price because I told myself that it was worth it.

I've met hundreds of musicians who suffered aches and pains because of the hours spent perfecting their art. Most had terrible posture—the first clue that a problem exists. How often do we see a dedicated musician with excellent posture? The two just don't seem to go together.

Knowing that I was used to discipline, my chiropractor advised me to take up yoga. My first class was a disaster. Accustomed to starring, I was humiliated by not being able to perform the simplest stretch. I asked for a private lesson to help me design an at-home practice.

Six weeks after practicing on my own at home, I joined another beginners' class. In the months that followed I developed a whole new attitude toward exercise. My whole life changed. Yoga gradually became an essential part of my focus—physically, intellectually, emotionally and therefore spiritually. That sounds intense, really overboard, like a new convert to some way-out religion, but I don't know how else to put it.

In school we learned how to play volleyball and other sports. We also did bouncing calisthenics, which can compact our bodies rather than lengthening them. In my earlier adult years I was busy raising three kids and performing on television. I figured I was getting enough exercise keeping up with daily life. What a common excuse that is! The fact is, even cars that are constantly driven and not maintained end up in a junkyard. That's where my neglected body was headed.

Now, five years later, yoga is as important to me as music. At 65, I'm more healthy and energetic by far than I was at 40, and to my delighted surprise I have been found worthy of sharing my yoga knowledge and experience with a beginning senior citizen class in my mobile home community.

By nature I'm hyper and highly energetic. Yoga provides a peaceful, tranquil place for me to just be. Stretching slows me down and makes patience possible. Yoga reminds me that there's no hurry to perfect a piece of music or write the final scene in a story. I will still be here tomorrow, and the music or story will benefit from me taking a breather.

My grown children, who are not as limber as I, can see me stretching farther and becoming stronger with every passing month. I can't help asking if I'm getting younger as they're growing older.

Jean Getchel:
Yoga Is Simply a Joy to Do

For all the reasons one can give for doing yoga, I would say first of all that it is simply a joy to do. One works with nature to create a calmness of spirit in a way that nothing else can duplicate. Yoga is also completely non-competitive and without negative impact on joints. Joints, instead, are made more flexible. Yoga is a gentle form of movement that greatly reduces injury, relieves stress as it develops concentration, builds strength, tones muscle, and helps develop balance.

I have had scoliosis, a lateral curvature of the spine, since my teenage years. Since discovering yoga, I have found that its practice has stopped the progression of the curve and has strengthened the muscles that help keep my spine as straight as possible.

I also had a stroke three years ago that briefly paralyzed my right side, leaving the muscles on that side weak. Yoga has helped to strengthen those muscles and to make me aware of the imbalances of the body so that I can work to correct them.

Eight

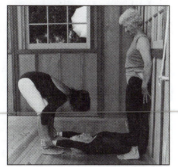

Yoga Techniques to Prevent or Overcome Arthritis

Just as a pebble produces ever widening concentric ripples on the surface of a still lake, the positive effects of a yoga practice spread into all aspects of one's life. As muscle strength, joint flexibility and neuromuscular coordination improve, one develops the ability to move with ease and confidence. This vitally important enhancement of mobility brings with it independence, self-determination and renewed interest in life. As exercise tolerance improves, yoga's salutary effects cascade into a positive, self-perpetuating cycle, replacing the pernicious negative cycle of inactivity, deterioration and depression.

—MARY PULLIG SCHATZ, M.D.
YOGA JOURNAL, MAY/JUNE 1990

Over 40 million Americans are struggling with arthritis. The term "arthritis" means "inflammation of the joints" and refers to a number of diseases that produce deterioration in various joint structures, which causes pain and immobilization. Severe arthritis often results in loss of function and deformity. In extreme cases, people who suffer with these diseases are no longer able to live independently. I have had personal experience assisting people with arthritis who were wheelchair-bound. I understand the extreme suffering involved in this disease.

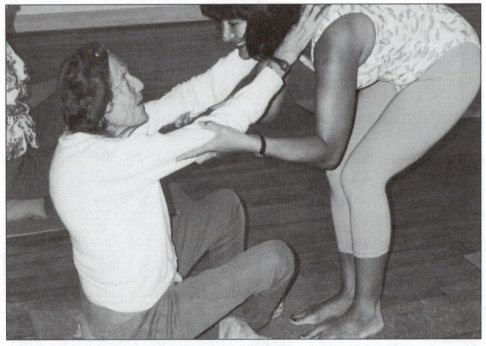

Students with painful arthritis often need special encouragement.

There are two main types of arthritis: osteoarthritis and rheumatoid arthritis. Rheumatoid arthritis is a chronic inflammatory disorder, resulting in stiffness in the joints and muscles, joint erosion and pain.

Osteoarthritis is a degenerative disorder that erodes the cartilage that cushions areas where bones rub against one another. The roughening of this normally smooth tissue makes moving difficult and painful. Osteoarthritis frequently occurs in people who are overweight or whose joints are painful from extreme overuse.

The cycle of arthritis begins with joint pain and swelling. As you probably know from even minor injuries, most of us respond to pain that occurs during movement by keeping still. However, we now know that one of the worst things for someone with arthritis is inactivity. Instead, regular gentle movement helps reduce pain and maintain mobility. Physicians are discovering that an appropriate yoga-based exercise program expands range of motion without stressing or straining joints.

To remain healthy, joints must move and bear weight. Without weight-bearing, bones become fragile and prone to fracture and collapse—the condition we call osteoporosis, discussed in chapter 7.

Physical movement promotes health in many systems of the body. Movement increases circulation which, in turn, reduces swelling and increases delivery of oxygen and nutrients to the joint tissues to facilitate their healing. With immobilization, a cycle of deterioration begins: muscles shorten from lack of stretching, which, in turn, creates deforming contractures. Unused muscles lose strength. This weakness, coupled with joint swelling, makes the joints unstable. Joints in this condition are vulnerable to dislocation, increased injury and pain. As arthritis patients feel weaker and more vulnerable, they become increasingly fearful and dependent; they feel tired and depressed.

Unlike other forms of physical exercise, yoga has something for everyone. No one is excluded. People with chronic disease and disabilities face "can't" at every turn in their lives: they can't play golf, can't play tennis, can't run, can't over-exert themselves, can't walk without canes, some can't walk at all. But everyone can do yoga. In yoga, there are no can'ts. Yoga can be modified and adapted to suit the needs of everyone.

—*Lorna Bell, R.N.*, Gentle Yoga, For People with Arthritis, Stroke Damage, Multiple Sclerosis and in Wheelchairs

Because movement is crucial to so many physiological processes, the arthritic person's health tends to deteriorate. The normal functioning of the immune system declines, infections and illnesses occur, and the person becomes frustrated and depressed. This cycle is self-perpetuating.

Generally, physicians advise regular gentle exercise for people with osteoarthritis because it tones muscles and reduces stiffness in joints. Yoga is an ideal form of exercise because its movements are fluid and adaptable. Moreover, students progress gradually, beginning with simple stretches and strengthening poses, and advancing to more difficult postures only as they become stronger and more flexible.

If necessary, you can begin yoga with gentle movements sitting in a chair or lying on the floor. Simple "one-joint" movements will gently loosen your joints and relax your muscles. These therapeutic yoga-based movements also improve your breathing and help relieve physical and emotional tension.

You can gradually add weight-bearing standing postures, with the help of a wall or table, wall ropes, chairs, blocks and other props described in chapter 3, to improve your strength, flexibility and balance. You can do standing postures holding on to a sturdy chair, wall or table, so that you'll feel safer and steadier. A regular exercise program is not only physically beneficial; it is extremely valuable psychologically because it increases your confidence that even though you have arthritis, you're not going to become a prisoner in a wheelchair.

Nellie Eder, an octogenarian yoga teacher who overcame arthritis with the help of yoga and proper nutrition, recommends self-massage and acupressure to help bring warmth and improved circulation to the joints. It is advisable to seek the services of a qualified massage therapist or other health professional familiar with holistic therapies to help you on your journey back to health.

I encourage you to seek the help of a teacher and to make yoga postures, breathing, relaxation and meditation techniques an important part of your daily routine. These techniques improve your respiration throughout the day as well, helping to relieve anxiety and pain. You can use yoga's breathing and relaxation techniques any time to relieve stress and tension. Remember that calm, slow, rhythmic breathing helps to release both physical and emotional tension by flooding the body and brain with oxygen. Remember, too, that the regular daily practice of deep relaxation—quieting the mind and body for even a few minutes at a time—is restorative to every cell of your body and encourages healing.

Arthritis need not mean a prognosis of inevitable disability. By practicing consistently, every day, you can reduce pain, build your strength and live with health and renewed energy.

Guidelines for a Yoga Program
for Arthritis

Yoga's approach to arthritis recognizes the interaction between the mind, body and spirit. Combining medical evaluation, nutrition, yoga, massage and other holistic therapies can break the debilitating cycle of arthritis. Yoga helps people with arthritis to be aware of their physical limitations without being paralyzed by them.

An intelligent, non-mechanical, individualized stretching and strengthening program is one of the keys to restoring health to arthritic joints. Properly aligned

> Moving hurts, but not moving destroys. Incorrect movement harms, but intelligent movement heals.
> —Mary Pullig Schatz, M.D.

movements designed to strengthen weak muscles and stretch those that have shortened are crucial to restoring stability and range of motion.

Keep the following tips in mind as you exercise:

- **Respect pain**. People with arthritis must learn the difference between the beneficial feeling of muscles stretching and the pain that signals harm. They must distinguish between the normal discomfort of moving stiff joints and the pain caused by a destructive movement or an excessive demand on a joint. Never bounce. Bouncing causes reflex tightening of muscles and can result in torn muscles and tendons. Sudden or severe pain is a warning. Continuing an activity after such a warning may cause joint damage. In general, if pain lasts more than two hours after an activity, ask someone who understands good alignment to check how you are practicing. If your alignment is good, consider easing up on your effort and experiment with holding those positions you suspect are causing pain for less time. Try moving more slowly and practicing more regularly. Most problems can be overcome by paying close attention to your body's innate feedback system.
- **Balance work and rest**. Conserve energy. Balance activity and rest. This principle applies to exercise as well as to daily activities. Overwhelming fatigue is counterproductive and may even be harmful. Weakened, fatigued muscles set the stage for joint instability and injury. Balance your active yoga session with yoga's deeply relaxing restorative poses. Restorative poses will help your internal healing processes to work.

- **Breathe properly**. Without fully expanding your lungs, the muscles you are exercising cannot be adequately supplied with oxygen. Holding your breath while stretching inhibits relaxation. Smooth, peaceful, rhythmic breathing through the nose reduces pain and tension and increases the feeling of deep relaxation that follows a stretching session.

- **Maintain muscle strength and range of motion**. Think about the way your body works, then use each joint in its most stable and functional anatomical plane. Avoid extending your limbs abruptly or in unnatural directions. Also, be careful not to hold a single position for too long. There is no set answer to the perennial question, "How long should I stay in the pose?" Long enough so that a healthy change has been made. Not so long that your body feels unhealthy strain or stiffens up from leaving muscles in a static position too long. Avoid mechanical repetitions and counting while exercising. Watch the flow of your breath and your body's response to a particular pose or exercise. Learn to tune into what your body is telling you.

- **To help maintain muscle strength and range of motion, learn to use yoga props**. Review the benefits of props in chapter 3. Remember, the more problems you are experiencing, the more useful yoga props are. Props allow you to hold poses longer so you can experience their healing effects. By supporting the body in a yoga posture, muscles can lengthen in a passive, non-strenuous way.

  The use of props helps improve blood circulation and breathing capacity. Props help you stretch, strengthen, relax or improve your body alignment.

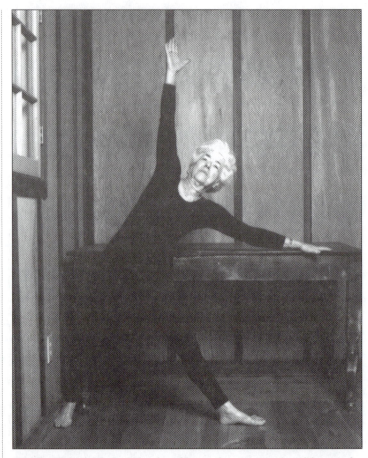

Standing poses with the help of a table or other prop can be a life-saver for people with arthritis.

By providing more height, weight or support, props help you extend beyond habitual limitations and teach you that your body is capable of doing much more than you think it can. This is especially important for people who are coping with arthritis.

Yoga props make postures safer and more accessible. People with arthritis may already be quite stiff by the time they start yoga. Props allow them to practice poses they would ordinarily have great difficulty in doing. Props help conserve energy and

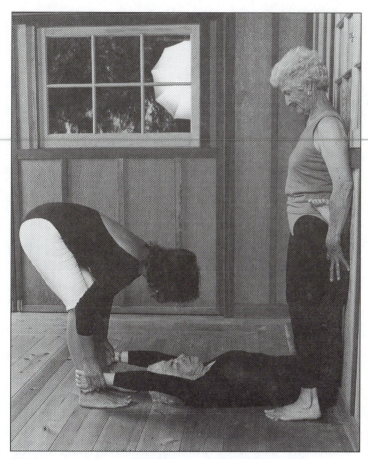

Helping a new student with stiff legs and shoulders to stretch.

allow people to practice more strenuous poses without overexerting themselves. Props are invaluable for people with arthritis, who must learn to exercise without strain and fatigue.

- **Warm up**. Although affected joints should be moved through a full range of motion at least once a day, it is unrealistic and possibly harmful to expect to attain full range of motion on the first try. Work into a pose gradually. It is often helpful to relax in a hot bath or shower before you practice.

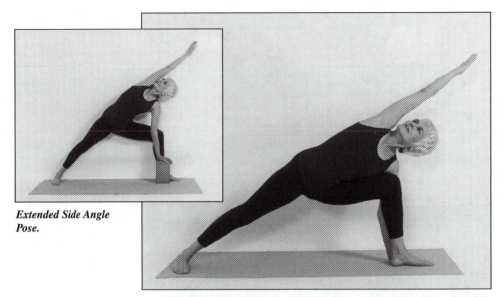

Extended Side Angle Pose.

Standing poses remove stiffness from the hips and knees. People with arthritis can practice against a wall and make the pose easier by using a block or chair for support.

• **Walk**. Walking is the ideal companion to an intelligent, therapeutic stretch-and-strengthen program. The tranquilizing effect of its moderate rhythmic exercise decreases pain. The movement and weight-bearing aspect of walking improves joint health. Equally important, walking can take you outdoors, in touch with nature, the greatest of all healers—uplifting to the mind and spirit. Pace yourself, walk where there are places to rest and stop there when you feel fatigued. Be in the moment and walk with awareness of the beauty around you.

Yoga for Arthritic Hips, Knees and Hands

The areas most commonly affected by arthritis are the hips, knees and hands. Like the knees, the hips often develop flexion contractures or are immobilized because tendons and muscles have shortened. These limit full straightening of the thigh at the pelvis. As a result, the hip joint frequently remains somewhat bent. With decreased movement, the muscles and soft tissues around the hip shorten, causing the joint space to decrease, and putting additional wear and tear on the gliding surfaces. If a person becomes more sedentary in an effort to minimize pain, bones and cartilage receive less weight-bearing stimulation. Bone spurs may even develop to further limit movement.

Prolonged pain and the natural impulse to immobilize the knee can cause flexion contractures, shortened muscles and tendons that immobilize the knee in a bent position. When muscles around the knee, including the front thigh muscles (quadriceps), shorten, this decreases the space in the joint.

Lack of exercise also weakens the thigh and calf muscles. Their strength provides stability and support for the knee. When the soft tissues of the joint swell, this causes compression and reduces space in the joint even further.

Standing poses such as the Right-Angle Pose are crucial for stretching out contractures and building supportive strength in the hip, buttocks and thigh muscles. Moving the head of the femur in the hip socket in the standing poses and in the range of motion exercise helps distribute synovial fluid, lubricating the joint's surfaces.

The same standing poses recommended for hips are also critical for knee rehabilitation. They provide stretching to relieve contractures, create more space in the knee joint for synovial fluid circulation, and develop the strength of the thigh and calf muscles to more adequately

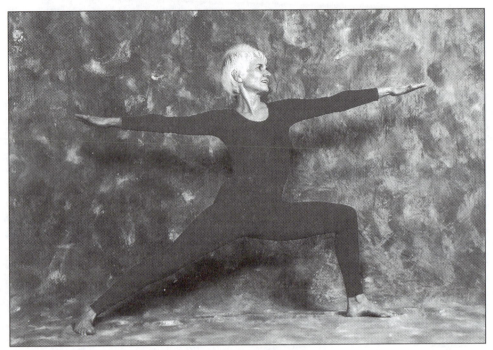

In the Right-Angle Pose, you feel supremely alert and confident.

support the knee. The psychological benefits of experiencing your own strength increase and stamina improve are also important. The ability to "stand on your own two feet" cannot be underestimated.

Modified
Hero's Pose

Modifying positions that require bent knees such as the Hero Pose, or *Virasana,* are important for gradually restoring flexibility in the front thigh muscles or quadriceps. Postures such as Virasana also initiate a squeezing action in the soft tissue of the knee, which helps reduce swelling. (Refer to chapter 5 for instructions.)

Yoga Stretching Positions for the Hands

When arthritis develops in the hands, their normal movements are altered and the fingers begin to slant outward toward the little finger side of the hand. As swelling over-stretches the joint-stabilizing structures, inflammation often causes dislocation in the joints. Frequently, the fingers and wrists become discolored and deteriorate. Sometimes muscular shortening makes it impossible to open the hand fully or to separate the fingers. Swelling in the wrist can cause pain and numbness in the hand (carpal tunnel syndrome).

In the following exercises, hands and wrists should not be placed in any position that accentuates or encourages deformity. Every movement should be designed to move the hand back toward normal.

Namaste (Prayer) Position

Sit or stand and press your palms together in prayer position. This position helps to stretch the muscles in the hand and straighten the fingers. If you have arthritic wrists or carpal tunnel syndrome, practice *Namaste* with forearms touching.

1. Gently press the palms and fingers of both hands together. As you breathe smoothly and evenly, encourage the fingers to move toward the thumb side of the hand. Hold for several breaths. Release the pressure but keep the hands together for a few more breaths. Then repeat the effort three or four times.
2. Gently, firmly and evenly press the palms together. Smoothly open the fingers and spread

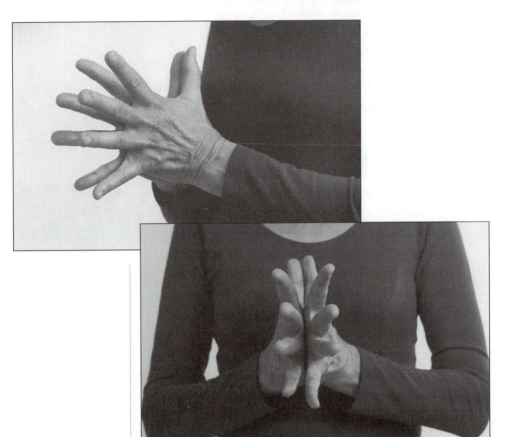

Stretching the hands in Prayer Position helps straighten the fingers.

them as wide as possible. Try to spread them evenly, moving them more and more toward the thumb side of the hand. Hold and stretch for a few breaths. Release and repeat.

3. Firmly and evenly press the palms together, especially the parts of the palm at the base of each finger. Stretch the fingers backwards, away from each other, gradually increasing the V-shaped space between them. Again encourage the fingers to move toward the thumb side of the hand. Encourage your fingers to stretch for three or four

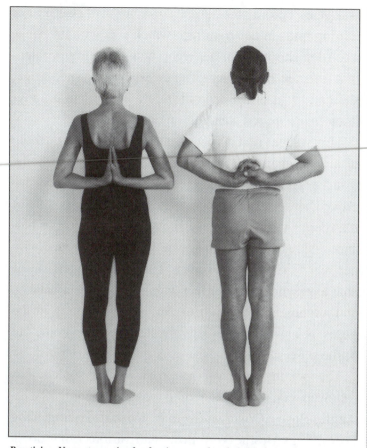

Practicing Namaste or simply clasping your hands behind your back improves your posture. These positions prevent stiffness in the hands and wrist.

more breaths. Release and repeat three or four more times.

One Student's Program for Arthritis in Knees and Hips

"I might be in a wheelchair or much worse, if not for yoga," said one 78-year-old student, who has been attending class two or three times a week for the last four years. Diagnosed with osteoarthritis in her knees two years before she started yoga, she had pain in her left hip, pins in her right hip (which was without pain), a left leg shorter than her right, and a hearing problem that affected her balance. When she first started yoga, she had to sit down or hold onto a support to do anything that required standing on one foot.

This student first started standing poses with the help of a wall, chair and wall ropes. She practiced at home using a kitchen counter or table. As her balance improved, she began to practice the poses in the middle of the room. At first, because she could not hold her balance and her legs and hips were stiff, she practiced with her feet fairly close together. Three years later, she is able to practice with her feet wide apart, and her balance and alignment are beautiful. She enjoys staying in the poses. In class she is usually the last person to come out of the pose.

The healing core of the program this student has followed consists of standing poses including Right-Angle Pose, Downward- and Upward-Facing Dog Poses, Legs-Up-the-Wall Pose, and various lying down and seated poses. During her first and second year of yoga, standing poses were most often practiced with her back on the wall, leaning into the wall and holding wall ropes. As her balance improved, she practiced near a wall for safety, but without depending on the wall. She now practices in the center of the room. She generally starts class by relaxing with her legs up the wall in various positions—legs straight up, legs wide apart, soles of the feet together and ankles loosely crossed. This legs-on-the-wall routine is followed by Child's Pose and Downward- and Upward-Facing Dog. Her most challenging position, kneeling in Hero Pose with a big bolster under her bottom and padding under feet, is generally practiced at the end of class. This student also enjoys practicing seated forward bends, Bridge Pose, floor twists, Shoulderstand-at-the-Wall and, most recently, Right-Angle Handstand.

Nellie Eder:
One Octogenarian Yoga Teacher's Experience
with Yoga and Arthritis

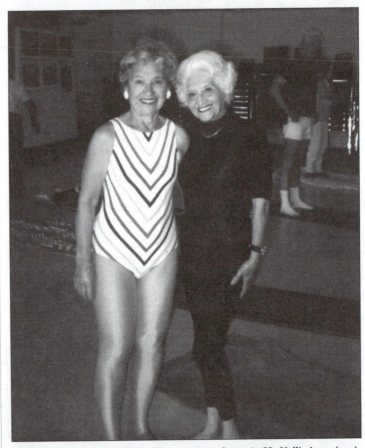

Nellie Eder (right), with one of her many students. At 89, Nellie is an inspiration to people of all ages.

Over the years I have met many people who started yoga as therapy for arthritis and who credit gentle stretching combined with chiropractic care, improved nutrition and an inner-body cleansing program, including juice fasting and colon hydrotherapy, for the recovery of their health. Nellie Eder, an 89-year-old yoga teacher in Palm Springs, California, turned to yoga when she was 50 to combat an advanced case of crippling rheumatoid arthritis that began in her early 30s.

"The pain was so bad," she told me, "I used to step outside and scream." Both her physical and social activities were severely curtailed by constant pain. Her doctors offered pain pills. By the time she reached 50, Nellie was in the advanced stages of arthritis and headed for a wheelchair.

At this time she became friends with a woman who introduced her to natural and holistic health concepts, which were not as widely recognized 35 years ago as they are now. Nellie said it gradually dawned on her that all the pain pills and other medications were killing her.

"This friend told me about yoga and a vegetarian diet," she continued. "I took all the pills and dumped them. I changed my diet and stopped eating meat and sugar. I also took colon hydrotherapy treatments and ate a cleansing diet of mainly fresh fruits and vegetables. I found that the yoga stretching benefited my body, and the accompanying meditation allayed my pain and enabled me to get complete control of my body."

Nellie has spent the past years teaching yoga at various senior centers. At one nursing home she met a 94-year-old woman who couldn't get out of a wheelchair. Nellie worked with her patiently and gently, showing her how to improve her breathing and stretch and strengthen her legs. According to Nellie, within three months the woman was walking without a cane.

This spirited octogenarian also teaches students how to do foot and hand reflexology (pressure-point massage therapy), which she feels is increasingly useful as we grow older. She believes elderly people need to explore natural, holistic, nutrition-oriented therapies instead of traditional medications.

After falling, fracturing her pelvis and severely spraining her sacroiliac joint, Nellie recently recovered her ability to walk. "At the hospital, the orthopedist told me, 'I'm sorry but you're not going to walk again.' 'Well,' I said, 'that's the second time in my life the doctors told me that I would never walk!'" To me, Nellie looks as if she could win a dance competition.

Nellie tells her students, "Don't come to me unless you practice every day. Nobody can help you unless you make up your mind to follow through."

Lolly Font:
Aging People Respond Beautifully to Yoga

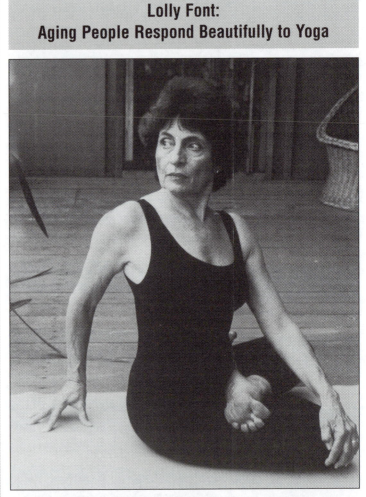

Lolly Font in Full Lotus Twist Pose.

Lolly Font is a teacher with an M.A. in Education. At 43, after raising five children, she became paralyzed with arthritis in her spine, neck, shoulders and hands. Yoga became her saving grace.

Obvious to me now but not then, I was in the process of a deep transformation. Miraculously, I discovered yoga, and I broke through the paralysis and stiffness in my body as the asana practice washed its magic through my being. Never an athletic person, I was overwhelmed by the beauty of the postures and the feelings of accomplishment and satisfaction I derived from attaining mastery over each pose. The expanded breathing, stretching, postural alignment and balance challenged my arthritic joints and created a new life for me.

Within four years my marriage broke up. This was not without pain. The pain in my joints and the pain in my heart were healed over a long tumultuous period of deepening practice.

Lolly went on to study at the Iyengar Yoga Institute in San Francisco, work with senior Iyengar teachers in the United States and Greece, and travel to India, where she studied with B.K.S. Iyengar. Afterward she earned a master's degree in transpersonal psychology and now does dreamwork. She and three partners began a yoga center. She is now a 70-year-old grandmother of eight and leads yoga retreats in Hawaii.

When I first trained as a yoga teacher, I asked for guidance in my daily meditation. I received a vision of a stooped, aging woman with a round back. At that moment I knew I had to teach seniors. I started a program for seniors at the Jewish community center. My students were my greatest teachers. They taught me about the effects of aging on older bodies and how yoga could reverse common problems. Learning by doing appeals to me and that is what I did.

Aging people are not touched very much, and they responded beautifully to the adjustments in the postures. Because they have lived in their bodies for a long time, they become unaware of subtle changes. When these subtleties multiply, they may expand into larger problems. I was able to point these physical problems out to them and help to avert or minimize some adverse outcomes. Maturing adults have physical problems such as difficulties with hands, feet, walking, eyesight, diet and sleep. In the yoga class they can discuss these problems and gain support from the teacher and the group. Moving together in a group also creates a pleasant social environment and encourages friendships among like-minded people outside of class.

Nine

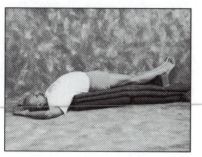

Opening the Heart with Yoga

Your Heart: Where Body, Mind and Spirit Converge

A lot of people swear by yoga—they love that more than anything else we do. It's another form of mindfulness, and it has the added benefit of reversing disuse atrophy and really toning the body. It's a full-body musculoskeletal strengthening and conditioning exercise. Yoga postures redirect the energy flow in your body and your mind. When you use yoga as a door into awareness of the body, it can teach you all sorts of things. You get to know your body on a totally intimate level. . . . When you're practicing yoga, you're releasing tension, and the tension isn't always in the body, it can also be in the heart, in the mind, or in feeling states. Release of that tension can put you back in touch with yourself on a very deep level. It's an inner experience of coming home.

—JON KABAT-ZINN, PH.D., INTERVIEW WITH BILL MOYERS IN *HEALING AND THE MIND*

Heart disease is the single most common cause of death in affluent countries like ours. In most Americans, heart disease is caused by a narrowing or blocking of the coronary arteries that deliver blood to the heart. The physical factors that contribute to heart disease—inherited risk factors, diabetes, high blood pressure, elevated serum cholesterol, deposits of plaque in the coronary arteries, smoking, poor diet, lack of exercise, job pressures, stress and other lifestyle-related considerations—explain only in part the cause of heart disease.

If the arteries are obstructed, blood flow is reduced, which reduces the amount of oxygen the heart receives and impairs its normal functioning. Yet heart disease is highly individual. Someone with relatively little obstruction in the coronary arteries can be incapacitated by angina, or squeezing chest pains, while another person with far more severely obstructed arteries may not be aware of any problem. Some people have run marathons with 85 percent of their coronary arteries blocked, while others with no sign of arteriosclerosis have dropped dead of a heart attack. It is clearly impossible to explain heart disease exclusively from physical causes.

Over 300 years ago, William Harvey, the founder of modern heart physiology, understood that the mind and emotions affect the health of the heart. "Every affection

Western techniques, such as drugs and surgery, can be very helpful in a crisis, but they are limited. . . . The stress management techniques derived from yoga address the more fundamental issues that predispose us to illness. And while yoga is a very powerful system of stress management, these techniques were designed for something much greater—as tools for transformation.

—*Dean Ornish, M.D.,*
Dr. Dean Ornish's Program for Reversing Heart Disease

of the mind that is attendant with either pain or pleasure, hope or fear," he said, "is the cause of an agitation whose influence extends to the heart."

In our era, Norman Cousins, after surviving a massive heart attack, wrote in *The Healing Heart*:

> *The human heart is not sealed off from countless processes that take place within the human body. It is a point of culmination, a collection center for all the malfunctions or deficiencies that exist in the body as a whole. It is a zone of infinite vulnerability to all the anguishes and insults and provocations of mind, soul and body.*

Dr. Dean Ornish's Prescription for Reversing Heart Disease

"Your heart is the place where your body, psyche and spirit all converge," writes Dean Ornish, M.D., in his book *Dr. Dean Ornish's Program for Reversing Heart Disease*. This famous and popular physician teaches that the health of the cardiovascular system involves all aspects of a human being—physical, emotional and spiritual.

Ornish's healthy lifestyle "prescription," which includes yoga postures and meditation, won the backing of mainstream medicine in the early 1990s, when one of the nation's largest providers of health insurance, Mutual of Omaha, announced that it would cover the $5,000-per-year cost of his program.

Ornish's program prescribes a low-fat vegetarian diet; yoga-based stress management techniques, including stretching, meditation, breathing and deep-relaxation techniques; a program to stop smoking; support-group

With tears and time you can heal any pain. Not doing so causes ill health and drains energy. Rage, hate and revenge are the biggest killers.
—*Elisabeth Kübler-Ross*

sessions; the development of communication skills; and directions for safe and moderate exercise.

His landmark research validates this holistic approach. After just one year on the program, his patients show a measurable reduction of blockages in their coronary arteries and sufficient relief from symptoms to make angioplasty or bypass surgery unnecessary.

In a *New Age Journal* interview, Dr. Ornish explains that:

> *Bypass surgery is much like clipping the wires to a fire alarm and going back to sleep while your house burns down, or like mopping up the floor around a sink that's overflowing without also turning off the faucet. It is now known that after five years, on the average, half of all the bypassed arteries have clogged up again, and within seven years, 80 percent have. And angioplasty, a newer technique in which a small balloon is inserted in the artery and then inflated to open blockage, doesn't fare any better. Within four to six months an estimated one-third have closed up again.*

In America, more money is spent on treating heart disease than any other illness—estimates range from $78 billion to $94 billion annually. More than $7 billion a year is spent on bypass surgery alone. When a doctor performs bypass surgery on a patient, the insurance company pays at least $30,000. If he or she performs a balloon angioplasty, the insurance company pays at least $7,500. If a doctor spends the same amount of time teaching that patient about nutrition and stress management, the insurance company pays considerably less.

Data/studies show that exercise and meditation can reverse the biological markers of aging—bone density, strength of muscles, blood pressure, aerobic capacity and others. It is now well-established that you can take a 97-year-old man or woman and put (him or) her on an exercise program and show reversals in the aging process. If people meditate regularly, their levels of DHEA—a hormone that usually declines with age—rise. Blood pressure drops, cholesterol levels balance, hearing and vision improve.

—*Deepak Chopra M.D.,*
Ageless Body,
Timeless Mind

The primary concept of Ornish's approach is that the farther back in the causal chain of events we can begin treating a health problem, the more powerful and lasting the healing will be. He describes how all the traditional risk factors—cholesterol, blood pressure, age, gender, genetics, smoking, diabetes, obesity, sedentary lifestyle, etc.—explain only half the reason some people get heart disease and others don't.

His nonsurgical, non-drug therapy, healthy-lifestyle approach to solving the great problem of heart disease has been endorsed by the American Heart Association and the President's Task Force on Health Reform. The "heart" of the program includes spending an hour a day practicing stretching and breathing exercises, deep relaxation and meditation. Ornish's program recognizes the importance of daily relaxation periods for preventing future heart deterioration. He recommends the practice of restorative yoga postures to ease stress and live a more balanced life.

Daily stretching, relaxation and meditation are crucial for people already suffering from high blood pressure and heart disease. Dr. Ornish and other health professionals who advocate the use of yoga techniques recognize that the course of heart disease is highly individual, and that our ability to overcome any health problem is greatly enhanced when we learn to consciously quiet and relax the mind and body.

> Yoga may be a centuries-old Eastern philosophy and art practiced by a variety of cultures, but it is also the finest, most adaptable form of combined physical and mental refreshment available today.
> —*Dawn Groves,*
> Yoga for Busy People

Chronic Tension and Heart Disease: The Fascinating Fight-or-Flight Response

Herbert Benson, M.D., coined the phrase "relaxation response" to describe the profound physical and mental

> If you think you can't spare 20 minutes a day for stretching and relaxing, I can almost guarantee that you are the very person that needs it the most!
> —*Judith Lasater, Ph.D.,*
> yoga teacher and author,
> Relax & Renew: Restful
> Yoga for Stressful Times

responses that occur when we consciously relax. According to Benson, the relaxation response is "a physiological state characterized by a slower heart rate, metabolism and rate of breathing, and lower blood pressure and slower brain-wave patterns." The opposite physiological response, characterized by a rapid heart rate, increase in blood pressure and quick, shallow breathing, is known as the "stress reaction" or "fight-or-flight response."

The fight-or-flight response is instinctual and deeply imprinted in our nervous system. It evolved to help us cope with immediate danger or situations of acute stress. Can you remember the last time you felt this reaction? All of us have experiences that trigger anger and anxiety.

By observing your own reactions to events in your life, you can become aware of your physical responses to emotions such as fear, anger and anxiety. When you are angry or anxious, your whole being becomes involved. Your breathing becomes rapid and shallow, to provide you with more oxygen either to do battle or run away. Observe how your muscles begin to contract. This is nature's way of preparing you to attack or protect yourself. Your metabolism and heart rate speed up, boosting your strength and energy. The amount of blood pumped with each heartbeat increases.

Next time you feel angry, see if you can feel your digestive system begin to shut down, so that more blood and energy can be diverted to the large muscles needed for fighting or running. If you are really angry, the arteries in your arms and legs begin to constrict and blood chemistry changes, so that clots form more quickly to conserve your blood should you be wounded.

According to heart and stress specialists, our bodies are designed to cope with acute stress, not the chronic stress of modern everyday life. When our survival mechanisms are chronically activated, they begin to exhaust our internal organs and nervous system. Arteries constrict not only in the arms and legs but also in the heart and brain. Blood clots are more likely to form inside the coronary and cerebral arteries, increasing blood pressure, sometimes leading to coronary thrombosis or stroke.

During emotional stress, our skeletal muscles constrict, causing pain and tension in the neck, back and shoulders. In addition, the internal smooth muscle lining the coronary arteries contracts, resulting in spasm in the heart muscle itself. Dr. Ornish describes the effect of chronic stress on the heart this way:

Under conditions of intense chronic stress, even the muscle fibers inside the heart itself can begin to contract so vigorously that the normal architecture of these fibers is disrupted, damaging the heart muscle. To me this is an amazing metaphor: The inability of the heart to relax causes the heart's muscle fibers to constrict to the point that it damages itself—like clenching your fist so hard and for so long that the bones and knuckles in your hand begin to break.

Obviously, stress reduction is not a luxury but a health-promoting and potentially life-extending technique. Begin now to become aware of your breath and take time to practice slow, calm, even breathing. It's the first step to feeling more relaxed.

Enlightenment: The Ultimate
Safeguard Against Stress

Yoga reverses the stress syndrome by bringing your body into the "relaxation response." However, ancient yogis and sages, wise men and women through the ages, have taught that the ultimate solution to stress is not simply learning how to manage it, but learning to see events in such a way that we don't create stress in the first place. Very often, the stress we blame on outer events is the product of our own emotions.

Coping with tension means understanding that stress comes not only from events in our daily lives but from how we react to them. We have all seen people who react entirely differently to the same situation: One will be very stressed while the other will just smile and say, "That's not important. I won't let it bother me." If you feel you are a person who increases the stress in your life emotionally, you may want to experiment with the way you see things. Altering your vision of events is sometimes a matter of simply reviewing priorities, examining what truly matters to you, or evaluating whether you will honestly care about whatever is bothering you a week, a month, or a year from now. Visual thinkers might draw a simple picture of the situation as they see it now, being sure to include a symbol of themselves, then moving the self step-by-step away from the center of the situation. How do they feel about it then? Positive habits of mind can be learned and practiced until we no longer feel at the center of the storm of daily life, but can observe, actively participate and remain at peace.

Practicing yoga is another way of finding your own

All religions encourage self-sacrifice, but when we are ill we pray to God to heal us. How inconsistent we are! To be simple, to appreciate what has been given to us, and to take care of our body, is an act of humility. . . . Do not fight your body. Do not carry the world on your shoulders like Atlas. Drop that heavy load of unnecessary baggage and you will feel better.

—*Vanda Scaravelli,*
Awakening the Spine

calm center. Gradually, as you discover the pleasure of sitting quietly or practicing the standing poses, you may realize that something has changed, that you feel a quiet joy and see a subtle shift in your perspective. As one of my students said, "It was like discovering an entirely new banquet of foods I had never experienced before." Because the practice of yoga unfolds gradually and is different each time, we can explore these subtle feelings and understandings throughout our lives. Until enlightenment comes, however, it helps to learn breathing, stretching and relaxation techniques for releasing mental and physical anxiety.

To understand the value and effect of relaxation techniques, keep in mind that tense, contracted muscles and shallow rapid breathing are major stress signals to the brain. If you can feel for yourself how during times of stress your entire sympathetic nervous system becomes stimulated (i.e., heart rate, blood pressure and muscular tension increase), you can more easily grasp how slowing down your breathing and stretching tense muscles sends out the opposite signal of relaxation, which not only calms and quiets the mind but relaxes the heart, balances your blood pressure, lowers cholesterol levels and helps to return all of the systems of the body to a healthier state.

Monday Morning Heart Attacks

"To be healthy, acknowledge the fact that if you try to take care of your health without taking care of what gives your life meaning, it's fighting the battle with one hand tied behind your back," says Larry Dossey, M.D., a specialist in mind/body medicine.

I believe the holistic healing systems of the future will combine the tremendous body of the "analyzed" knowledge of the traditional medical profession with the "synthesized" knowledge of the higher body/energy systems. The future holistic healing systems will diagnose and prescribe healing for all the energy bodies and physical body simultaneously as needed by the patient and incorporate both the inner and the outer healing processes. Medical doctors, chiropractors, homeopaths, healers, therapists, acupuncturists, etc. will all work together to aid the healing process.

—Barbara Ann Brennan,
Hands of Light:
A Guide to Healing
Through the Human
Energy Field

You can treat blood pressure, stop smoking, get your cholesterol level down—and do those things perfectly—but that is not covering the bases. We know that most Americans under the age of 50 who have their first heart attack have none of these major risk factors present. They check out fine! That's a way of saying that the meaningless, purely physical approach can't account for even a simple majority of first-time heart attacks.

Dr. Dossey's books eloquently challenge the most ingrained assumptions of modern medicine, such as the notion that the body is a machine; that it is fully automatic; that thoughts, attitudes and feelings are of little consequence; that consciousness is simply the product of chemicals in the brain; that there is nothing higher than the brain mechanism; that when the body dies, that is the end of it.

According to leaders in the field of mind/body healing, medicine rests on a set of assumptions that, when examined from a philosophical or scientific point of view, become extremely shaky. As Dossey says, most of us plod along without ever examining the fundamental questions about our life and health.

One fascinating signal that told him we ought to be looking at health from many angles is the Monday morning heart attack phenomenon. In the United States, more people have heart attacks on Monday morning between 8 and 9 A.M. than any other time. In a study done in the early 1970s, Dossey determined that the best predictor of heart attack was none of the major risk factors—not smoking, high blood pressure, diabetes or cholesterol—it was level of job satisfaction. In his book,

Meaning and Medicine, he asks, "What is the meaning of a person's job to them? What does a job represent or symbolize in their mind? Without bringing in meaning, we can't understand the origin of the most common killer in our society: heart disease."

Dossey claims that one of the first steps toward health is to simply acknowledge and honor the fact that we need to perceive our lives as meaningful, feel that our efforts are worthwhile and understand that even our illnesses have meaning. "Then you can go from there. It's impossible to spell out in any one person's life, what might follow. How should one person sort out their meanings?"

Can you imagine going for a free cholesterol check-up and having a medical technician ask you whether or not you're happy with your life? It's much easier to focus on cholesterol and blood pressure or to treat heart attacks when they occur. A doctor has a tough enough time getting a patient to exercise, eat right and cover all the physical bases. Nonetheless, as challenging as it is to examine ourselves mentally, emotionally and spiritually, the whole field of psychoneuro-immunology is demonstrating that thoughts are not simply ethereal notions that pass through the brain. Apparently our thoughts penetrate the body and affect every major system in the body—particularly the cardiovascular and immune systems—as much as, or even more than, food and exercise.

Scientific research continues to affirm the value of disciplines such as yoga. One of the most effective ways to lower cholesterol levels is simply to sit down twice a day for about 20 minutes and clear and quiet the mind. Cholesterol levels drop by about one-third. Dr. Dean Ornish says, "Even a few minutes of meditation a day brings real benefits."

How Posture Affects the Health of Your Heart

Notice how you are sitting as you read this. Don't change anything, simply observe yourself. Now deliberately slump forward as much as you can until you feel your internal organs pressing in on each other. How are you breathing now and how do you feel? These observations tell you how your everyday posture—the way you sit, stand and walk—affects your respiration, circulation and the health of your heart. Chronic slouching decreases circulation to all your vital organs.

When the chest is collapsed, your diaphragm barely moves down as you inhale. This keeps you from completely filling your lungs. It prevents the "chest pump" from helping to return blood to the heart. If the abdomen and chest are compressed most of the time, the lymphatic vessels, arteries and veins serving the vital abdominal organs may collapse, even partially. This reduces the circulatory cleansing of all these tissues, and minimizes the transportation of vital nourishment to the cells and the circulation of important hormones that regulate the body's processes. This compromises overall health, including the health of the heart.

One of yoga's most immediate effects is a dramatic improvement in our posture. People of all ages sigh with relief as the chest opens and they can breathe freely. For those with rounded shoulders and chronically stooped posture, basic standing poses begin to open the chest and expand the breathing process. More vigorous poses such as Upward and Downward Dog, both from the floor and stretching back and forth with wall ropes, further stretch the muscles of the front of the body, expand the chest and increase breathing capacity, as well as strengthen the back, chest and shoulder muscles.

Gentle supported backbends and various restorative postures expand the chest, lungs and rib cage without effort. These passive poses are useful for everyone, but are especially recommended after healing from heart surgery, and should be practiced with the guidance of a qualified instructor.

Breathing Freely, Relaxing Deeply Reduces Stress

Note in the photo on page 246 how the folded blankets positioned evenly under the back of the head and length of the spinal column, open and expand the chest, allowing the body to breathe freely and deeply relax.

All body/mind disciplines teach that the breath is a bridge between the body and the mind. Most present-day stress reduction techniques are based on this recognition. Conscious, calm breathing is one of the simplest, yet most elegant and effective ways to combine awareness of our physical body with consciousness of our mental and emotional state. Breathing is also a powerful means of relaxing your sympathetic nervous system, which governs the stress response, and accessing the healing effects of your parasympathetic nervous system, which governs the relaxation response.

Being aware of your breath and softly, calmly, regulating it in the way that I describe next sends a direct message of relaxation to the mind and nervous system.

The following technique comes from the teachings of B.K.S. Iyengar. It can be practiced either sitting upright or lying down. Even though the four steps look very

Breathing is the essence of yoga. Breathe naturally, without forcing. No pressure, no disturbance, nothing should interfere with the simple, tide-like movement of our lungs, as we breathe in and out. . . . Breathing is the most important part of our yoga practice.
—*Vanda Scaravelli,*
Awakening the Spine

simple, I recommend that you read the instructions all the way through at least twice before you begin. Note that what makes this way of breathing different from our usual, habitual way of breathing is the pause at the end of each exhalation.

Breathing to Calm the Mind and Reduce Stress

1. Inhale slowly, gently, without strain, through your nose.
2. Exhale slowly, gently, without strain, through your nose.
3. Pause briefly without straining or attempting to hold your breath.
4. Repeat steps 1, 2 and 3. Continue breathing in this calm, simple way for several minutes.

To review: at the end of every exhalation, pause without straining for a second or two before inhaling again. By pausing briefly after each exhalation, you may notice a spontaneous, natural, unforced continuation of the exhalation. This additional release of the breath completes a true, normal exhalation. In our habitual way of breathing, especially if we are tense, the exhalation is incomplete. We start each exhalation without allowing the previous exhalation to come to its natural conclusion. If you practice this new way of breathing regularly, your breathing will deepen naturally, effortlessly, and you will find yourself feeling calmer and more relaxed, even under what once seemed like stressful circumstances.

In daily life, practice watching your breath. As you observe its flow, inhale and exhale calmly through your nose. Do not try to impose a deeper breath on your natural breathing rhythm. By being aware of your breath and pausing without strain after each exhalation, you will feel a natural urge to inhale more deeply and freely. Follow this urge, without straining or forcing, and then return to normal breathing. Remember to practice this relaxed way of breathing whenever you want to calm down and relax—when stuck in traffic, while waiting in line or at the doctor's office, whenever you feel anxious or upset.

When lying down to relax, close your eyes and look down toward your heart. Allow your eyes to relax. Looking downward toward the chest helps your brain to relax. To help you relax further, cover your eyes, using an eyebag, if available (see the Resources section) or a damp folded facecloth. The gentle pressure of a light weight over the eyes reduces their involuntary movements and releases tension in the eyes and forehead.

When using folded blankets or pranayama (breathing) pillows to support your body, as described in the prop chapter, note how the shape of the blankets expands and opens the chest, and supports and encourages the natural curves of the spine. The body generally responds with delight and a sigh of relief upon being positioned on folded blankets or long, firm pillows. I consider their use absolutely essential for learning to breathe freely and relax deeply.

Some Facts About Breathing

- Changes in your body affect your breathing. When you walk or run uphill or otherwise exert yourself, your oxygen requirements go up and you breathe faster and deeper.

- Changes in your mind affect your breathing. If you are anxiously anticipating the dentist's drill, or about to deliver a speech, your breathing is apt to be rapid and shallow. Conversely, when you are sitting on a hill watching a sunset, getting a massage or petting your dog, you are more likely to breathe slowly and deeply.
- Changes in your breathing affect your body. Athletes, martial artists, singers, dancers and gymnasts all use breathing techniques to improve their performances.
- Changes in your breathing affect your mind. When you are worried, a few deep breaths can help calm you down. Deep breathing wakes up a tired mind.
- Changes in your posture dramatically affect your breathing. It is impossible to breathe deeply and freely if you slump.

There are many books and schools of thought on breathing techniques for reducing stress. The first step is to have the presence of mind to notice the way you breathe in both relaxed and tense situations. I believe that any changes made in breathing should be gentle and very gradual. When experimenting with deepening your breath, the rules are: Stop if you feel any strain, and inhale and exhale naturally for several cycles before you begin again. Remember to close your lips softly and breathe through your nose.

Stress and the Immune System

Stress depletes the body's reservoirs of vital energy. Stress also tends to speed up our metabolism to the point that even when we do have a chance to slow down and recuperate, we find we are unable to unwind and

> My regimen is targeted specifically to stress. Stress ages you. Yoga and meditation help me connect with my inner-self rather than my tensions. This is not to downplay calisthenics, weights and aerobics. But I know for a fact that they don't help my state of mind, or help my skin glow in quite the same way yoga and meditation do.
>
> —Raquel Welch

relax. Many people, as they are introduced to yoga's deep relaxation practices, discover that their bodies and minds need to re-learn what it feels like to experience a deep level of relaxation.

A potentially life-saving principle to remember is: The way you react to stress influences immunity more than the severity of the actual stressful event. Of the personality traits associated with low resistance to illness, feelings of helplessness are the most destructive. Just knowing that you can do something constructive when life seems overwhelming boosts your immune system. Even if the actual situation cannot be changed, reducing the body's reaction to stress by practicing relaxing yoga positions and peacefully observing the breath allows the mind and body to break the stress cycle, recuperate, and restore equilibrium.

EDITOR'S NOTE: *For further information on Dr. Dean Ornish's program for reversing heart disease, other resources and educational opportunities please write: The Preventive Medicine Research Institute, 900 Bridgeway, Suite 1, Sausalito, CA 94965, 415-332-2525.*

Alice Stevens:
Maturing at a More Satisfying Pace

Alice Stevens is a yoga instructor for the American Heart Association. She also teaches cardiopulmonary resuscitation (CPR) as part of a cardiac rehabilitation program. Unfortunately, she says, these days more and more young men and women are becoming afflicted with heart disease.

Yoga has enhanced my strong qualities, made me more aware of my not-so-hot ones, and helped me mature at a more satisfying pace. It takes a lot of energy and good spirits to thrive in a busy and happy life.

Older students sometimes need more encouragement until their confidence perks up and they start enjoying themselves in class. So many women and men who are older come into class for a whole new physical adventure, and I want it to be a good experience for them. At first they are easily intimidated, but once they begin to feel at home and the poses become familiar, they get stronger. It's wonderful to see them bloom.

I have found that the Downward-Facing Dog is the best pose in yoga for older students to regain or build posture, upper-body strength, flexibility, and to stretch those concrete hamstrings. I just love it when an elegant matron proudly tells me that she's teaching her husband the Dog Pose so he'll stand up straight.

Ina Marx:
If Your Life Has Purpose You
Can Never Grow Old

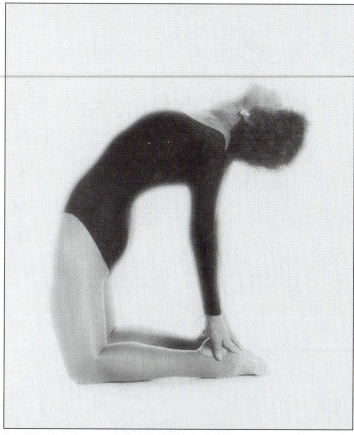

Ina Marx enjoys an exhilarating stretch in the Camel Pose.

Ina Marx, 76, is the author of Yoga and Common Sense *and* Fitness for the Unfit. *After an accident that left her severely disabled, she made a personal commitment to yoga.*

My own uphill climb began at age 40. I was totally devoid of self-confidence. Self-love and self-realization were not in my dictionary. I had struggled along with limited capacities for most of my life, plodding along as best I could. My life seemed a never-ending series of personal tragedies.

When I was 30, I was working in a luxury resort on weekends while my husband stayed home, taking care of our young daughter. I stayed overnight in a ramshackle firetrap reserved for the hotel's help. I was pregnant again as well. One night, as the staff members were sleeping, a fire broke out. I was in a room on the third floor, where many of us were trapped as flames spread and consumed the wooden staircase.

What saved me were my instincts. The only way to escape was through the window. There were two in the dormitory. One was always stuck and the other was blocked by a crowd of other panic-stricken occupants. I smashed the window that would not open. When the flames came unbearably close, I jumped, plummeting onto a concrete drive. By the time the fire truck arrived, the building had burned to the ground and 10 people were dead.

I had fractured my back and pelvis, cracked ribs and sustained internal injuries. My psyche was broken as well. I lost my unborn baby. First I was placed in a body cast. Later I graduated to a steel corset, which I was told I would wear for the rest of my life. Because I was in constant pain, I became addicted to tranquilizers, barbiturates, painkillers and three packs of cigarettes a day. I suffered from fatigue, insomnia and obesity. I spent all my time seeing a succession of physicians and physical therapists. Life held no meaning for me and I often contemplated suicide.

After two suicide attempts, I sought psychiatric treatment. I began to function better but broke down again. I found a new therapist and my mental attitude improved. Physically I was still a wreck, but decided to hang in there and try every healing method I heard of. One day someone said, "Try yoga!" I latched onto it as a last resort. At first, it seemed hopeless. I could not bend in any direction. However, I was determined to stick to it because I had caught a glimpse of a more hopeful future.

Discipline and hard work were the keys, and consistency was the vital factor. I didn't turn my whole life over to yoga, for I still had my family to take care of, but I practiced conscientiously for at least one hour each day. My back grew stronger. After three months I threw away my corset. My figure improved, I was healthier and more energetic. For the first time in years, I fell asleep easily. I gradually eliminated the tranquilizers and barbiturates that had been a staple in my diet. Quite naturally and painlessly, I gave up smoking.

As my body changed, so did my mental outlook. My sense of values changed as well as my attitude toward people. I developed more patience, kindness and tolerance. At age 40, I realized that I am responsible for my state of being and that I could attain any goal I desired.

I refused to be defeated by the laws of probability and defied the medical advice, "You must learn to live with your pain." I disproved the orthopedist's prescription, which would have confined me to a wheelchair for life. Although my back injuries have knitted, subsequent examinations have shown deterioration of several discs and a congenital curvature of my spine. Those who view my X rays find it incomprehensible that I can even walk. Yet my back is strong, supple and free of pain.

According to medical and societal standards, I am old. If I applied for a life insurance policy or a job, I would probably be rejected. But I maintain that age is irrelevant. I feel younger, healthier, am stronger, have more energy, vitality and optimism than I did in my earlier years. While I do not follow the popular expectations for aging, neither do I yearn for youth. There is no way to escape forever the exterior signs of aging. Old age, however, is a state of mind that can be changed. If your life has a purpose, you can never grow old.

Robert Whiteside:
Agile at 80, Nimble at 90

Robert Whiteside is author of Agile at 80, *a short, motivational book encouraging older adults to exercise, eat right and keep a fresh outlook on life.*

I think that one of the things people most dread and fear about old age is aches and pains, or being wheelchair-bound, a burden to themselves and others.

I myself and many others have demonstrated that such a fate is not necessary, if one follows nature's laws through proper nutrition, exercise and a positive mental attitude.

I'm an octogenarian now and still jog three miles before breakfast and play tennis a couple times a week. I also carry out an active professional career—traveling a third of the time.

If I were to write my book over again (I am shooting for *Nimble at 90*), I would emphasize yoga even more, and also more use of fresh vegetable juices.

Traces of old injuries pop up if I don't behave myself and each day remember to practice my yoga exercises to keep everything supple and in its proper place. It's marvelous what the human body will do, given half a chance.

The wisdom of the body—knowing how to sound alarms, receive supplies, do repairs, strengthen muscles, heal cuts, join a broken bone together—makes the best computer archaic.

Once you get started it's an upward spiral. Don't be ashamed of beginning modestly, but *do* begin. And do not get discouraged if some emergency keeps you from your whole program. Just do as my yoga instructor advises: start the next day where you left off.

Any time you are tempted to quit, consider the alternative. As my son-in-law quips, "It's better to be over the hill than under the hill!"

Ten

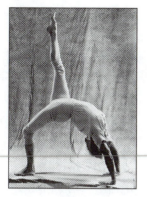

Backbends Open Posture, Lift Spirits and Expand Perspective

The intention, the long term goal, is to become completely fluid, completely liquid and sinuous. As I get older I'd like to be that. I'd like to have explored the entire range of my body's abilities. It's not that I'm afraid of getting old. I just want to get old in a certain way. I want to get old gracefully. I want to have good posture, I want to be healthy, and I want to be an example to my children.

—STING, INTERVIEWED BY GANGA WHITE,
IN *YOGA JOURNAL*, NOV/DEC 1995

*P*eople who just talk about, read books on, and go to lectures on spiritual matters are, to use my favorite analogy for this, much like the person who wants to learn to swim before getting into the water. Obviously, you must get into the water in order to discover that it can be trusted to hold you up; only then is learning to swim possible. . . . Practicing is the getting into the water—the acting on, rather than only listening to or talking and reading about spiritual matters. . . . You must act—practice.

—GEORGE JAIDAR, *THE SOUL: AN OWNER'S MANUAL, DISCOVERING THE LIFE OF FULLNESS*

Health is freedom. . . . As the sun opens the flowers delicately, unfolding them little by little, so the yoga exercises and breathing open the body during a slow and careful training. When the body is open, the heart is open. There is a transformation in the body's cells. They work in a different way and a new growth is possible.
—*Vanda Scaravelli,* Awakening the Spine

Backbends counteract many of the changes often considered to be a normal part of the aging process. As we grow older, the spine degenerates and we become shorter. Roundness of the upper back, known as kyphosis, is so common in older people in this culture that it is almost accepted as an inevitable part of the process of aging. As the back curves forward, the chest sinks, the lungs are at least partially compressed, and respiration is compromised. This has a negative impact on every system of the body, especially the cardiovascular system.

Bending backwards counteracts all of these tendencies. To breathe freely, we must release the tension in our chest, the chest cavity must be able to expand fully, and the muscles surrounding the rib cage must be free to stretch. Backbends free the chest, open the rib cage and encourage healthy breathing. After a series of backbends the whole body becomes charged with oxygen, making us feel exceptionally energetic and alive.

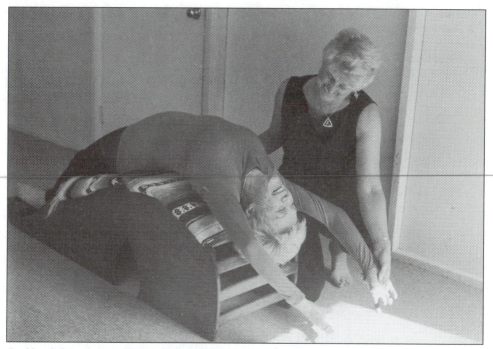

Backbends bring greater blood supply to the discs and nerves of the spinal column.

Backbends strengthen and refresh the entire body. Gently and gradually arching the body backwards lengthens and tones the entire spinal column, opens the shoulder joints, stretches the surrounding muscles, tendons and ligaments, and stimulates production of synovial fluid, the lubricant in the joints. Calcium deposits, bursitis and the general tension many of us carry in the upper back, neck, shoulders and arms can be relieved with backbends. Weight-bearing, active backbends also strengthen the arms, wrists and legs and increase circulation to the organs in the pelvis. In addition, backbends massage the kidneys and adrenals and stretch and stimulate the liver.

During a backbend, the front of the body is stretched to the maximum, especially the chest area. The opening of the chest opens the heart center. Backbends relieve

Whatever is flexible and flowing will tend to grow, whatever is rigid and blocked will wither and die.

—Tao Te Ching

depression by dispelling the heavy-hearted feeling we have when we are sad. Stretching backwards lifts your spirits, changes your perspective and makes both the mind and body feel light and free.

Begin practicing backbends gradually. If you are stiff, never force a backbend; instead, prepare the body by working on standing poses and practicing gentle supported backbends. As always, use common sense. You don't start a yoga stretching program with backbends any more than you would hike uphill 15 miles if you hadn't taken a long walk in many years. If you have back problems such as degenerative disk disease, or if you have high blood pressure, a history of stroke or heart trouble or other serious illness, do not attempt the more strenuous backbends without the guidance of a qualified teacher. Also, do not practice backbends during pregnancy.

Bridge Pose to Strengthen the Back (Setu Bandha Sarvangasana)

This pose is frequently prescribed by chiropractors and other doctors as part of a back-strengthening program. It is most effective done slowly and thoroughly, with yoga awareness of the breath, rather than repeated mechanically. Like Downward-Facing Dog and standing poses, it should be part of a core program for those who begin yoga after 50.

This pose can be done after standing poses or as part of a lying-down-on-the-floor series. For experienced students, it is safe preparation for more active, advanced backbends. Almost everyone of any age can enjoy doing the Bridge Pose from the first days of their practice.

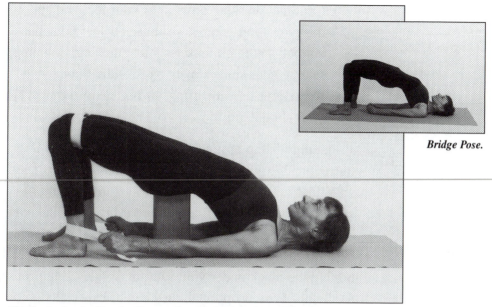

Bridge Pose.

This beginning backbend will strengthen the back and open the chest.

1. Lie on the floor or sticky mat, your knees bent, feet placed hip-width apart, fairly close to your bottom.

2. Relax in this position, watching your breath, allowing your belly to soften and relax. Wait until you feel your abdomen drop (a pleasant, relaxed, hollow feeling), and the back of your waist drop to the floor as your lower back releases and lengthens. Anchor the soles of your feet to the floor, turning your toes in slightly.

3. When you feel relaxed, tuck your tailbone under, toward your heels. Continue drawing your tailbone under, until your bottom naturally begins to lift off the floor.

4. Keeping your feet in line with your hips, press down into your feet even more and continue to slowly lift as much of your spine off the floor as you comfortably can.

5. Continue pressing down into your feet and stay in the pose long enough so that you feel your back, buttock and thigh muscles strengthening. Exhaling, release your spine slowly back to the floor.

6. Relax and repeat, lifting up higher to the tops of your shoulders.

Placing a strap around your feet and knees, as illustrated on the previous page, will remind you to keep your feet active, pressing firmly into the ground, and your knees parallel, in line with your hips. A block can be placed as shown by bringing your toes close to your bottom, lifting your pelvis high up and carefully positioning the block under your sacrum. While using props for Bridge Pose is optional, they can be especially helpful for beginners over 50.

Gentle Supported Backbends Create Breathing Space

Healthy circulation and respiration are fundamental to good health. Backbends, like many other yoga postures, stimulate and strengthen these two vital systems, which nourish, cleanse and invigorate the entire body.

The gentler, passive, supported backbend positions, practiced by lying over bolsters, stacks of folded blankets or yoga props such as the backbending bench in the photo on page 209, can generally be safely practiced by people with high blood pressure, heart disease, breathing difficulties and other stress-related problems. In fact, for such people these postures are especially beneficial.

Backbends make breathing easier by opening the rib cage and passively stretching and lengthening the chest muscles.

The young, the old, the extremely aged, even the sick and the infirm obtain perfection in Yoga by constant practice. Success will follow him who practices, not him who practices not. Success in Yoga is not obtained by the mere theoretical reading of sacred texts. Success is not obtained by wearing the dress of a yogi or a recluse, nor by talking about it. Constant practice alone is the secret of success. Verily, there is no doubt of this.

—*Hatha Yoga Pradipika*,
1:64-66

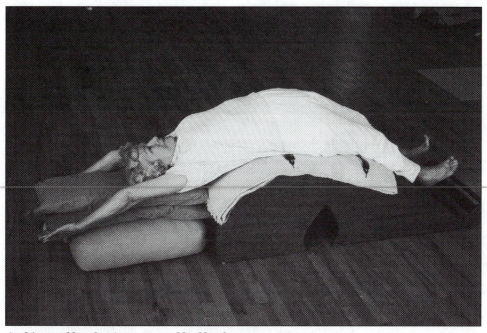

An 84-year-old student in a supported backbend.

Both the more strenuous active backbends and the gentler, passive backbend positions stretch the abdominal organs and expand the space in which they function, as well as improve blood supply to the area. When the body is placed in a passive supported backbend, muscles stretch, the chest and rib cage open, and breathing becomes easier, eliciting the soothing, restorative relaxation response.

To further understand the value of supported backbends, consider the changes that occur in our respiratory system after years of poor posture aggravated by emphysema, asthma or other breathing difficulties. When the chest is collapsed in the presence of lung disease, the lungs lose their normal elasticity, so it takes more muscular effort to move air in and out. If the chest is closed, tense and tight, and breathing is difficult, the muscles of the neck and shoulders (not meant for this purpose) are recruited to keep us breathing at least enough to keep the body alive.

When posture is chronically poor and the head is held forward, the upper back rounded, the neck and shoulder muscles are always partially contracted. In this chronic state of tension, the neck, shoulder and upper-back muscles require more oxygen and energy at the same time as their blood supply diminishes. Lactic acid builds up in the tissues, causing the muscles to become sore and stiff and respiration to be further restricted.

The body constantly monitors blood pressure, blood oxygen levels and muscle tension. Shallow breathing reduces the amount of oxygen available to tissues and cells. When the muscles are also chronically tense, the body interprets these signals to mean it is in a state of emergency and responds with the "stress response" discussed in chapter 9. Supported backbends counteract and reverse all of these postural and respiratory problems by deeply relaxing the muscles and opening the chest and rib cage. As muscular tension is released, circulation improves. The deep relaxation that takes place when one remains in a supported backbend, even for a short period, is healing and rejuvenating for the whole body.

Study the photo of Supported Bridge Pose on the following page and note how the support under the back and legs is placed end-to-end to accommodate the length of the body. The height of the support under your body depends on the length of your torso and the flexibility of your back. New students can begin with one or two single-fold blankets and gradually increase the height. Six to 12 inches in height works well for most people. Taller people can add height to the bolsters with one or

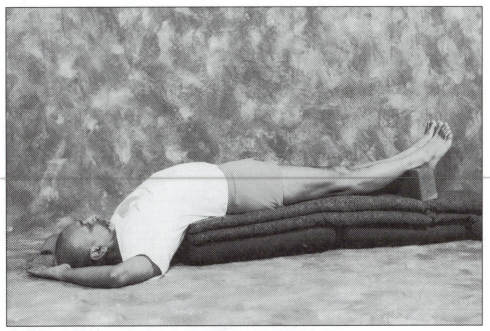

Yoga teacher Ramanand Patel demonstrates Supported Bridge Pose.

more blankets on top of the bolsters. You can also place a block under your heels, as illustrated. For details on practicing Supported Bridge Pose, review chapter 6, page 137.

B.K.S. Iyengar:
It Is Never Too Late to
Practice Yoga

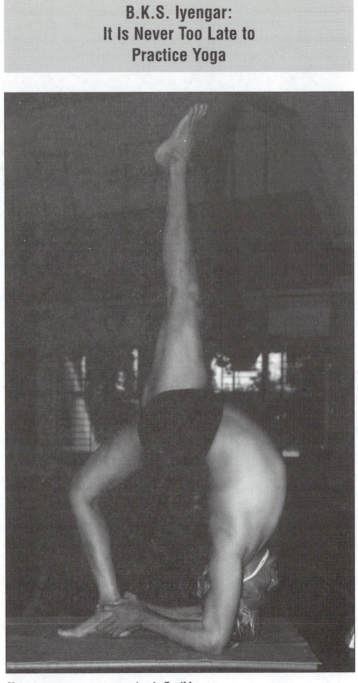

You are as young as your spine is flexible.

B.K.S. Iyengar, born December 12, 1918, is one of this century's foremost exponents of yoga. The author of Light on Yoga, Light on Pranayama, The Tree of Yoga *and many other books, Iyengar still performs a rigorous daily yoga practice that would challenge anyone at any age.*

It is never too late in life to practice yoga. If it were, then I should have stopped my practice long ago. Why should I do so now? Many Indian yogis reach a certain point in their lives and say they have reached *samadhi* [the highest state of spiritual evolution], so they don't need to practice any more. But I have not said that up to now. Why not? Learning is a delight, and there are many delights to be obtained through the practice of yoga. But I am not doing it now for delight! In the early days delight was the aim, but now it is a by-product. The sensitivity of intelligence which has been developed should not be lost. That is why the practice has to continue.

If you have a knife which you do not use, what happens to it? It gets rusted, does it not? If you want to go on using it, you have to sharpen it regularly. With regular sharpening you can keep it sharp forever. Similarly, having experienced samadhi once, how do you know that you are going to remain alert and aware forever? How can you say that you can maintain it without practice? You may forget and go back to enjoying your life in the same way as you did before. Can a dancer or concert performer give a fine performance if they have not practiced for a year? It is the same for a yogi. Though one may have reached the highest level, the moment one thinks one has reached the goal and that no practice is required, one becomes unstable. In order to maintain stability, practice has to continue. Sensitivity requires stability. It has to be maintained by regular practice.

You may be 50 years old, or 60 years old, and ask yourself whether it is too late in life to take up yoga practice. One part of the mind says, "I want to go ahead," and another part of the mind is hesitating. What is that part of the mind which is hesitating? Perhaps it is fear. What produces that fear? The mind is playing three tricks. One part wants to go ahead, one wants to hesitate and one creates fear. The same mind is causing all three states. The trunk is the same, but the tree has many branches. The mind is the same, but the contents of the mind are contradictory. And your memory also plays tricks, strongly reacting without giving a chance to your intelligence to think.

Why is an old man fond of sex? Why does his age not come to his mind at all? If he sees a young girl, his mind will be wandering, even though he may have no physical capacity. But ask him to do a little yoga, or something to maintain his health, "Oh, I am very old," he says. So the mind is the maker and the mind is the destroyer. On one side the mind is making you and on the other side the mind is destroying you. You must tell the destructive side of the mind to keep quiet—then you will learn.

Fear says that as you get older, diseases and suffering increase. Your mind says you should have done yoga earlier, or you should have continued and not stopped in your youth. Now you say you are very old and perhaps it is too late, so you hesitate. It is better just to start, and when you have started, maintain a regular rhythm of practice.

At a certain age the body does decay, and if you do not do anything, you are not even supplying blood to those areas where it was being supplied before. By performing asanas we allow the blood to nourish the extremities and the depths of the body, so that the cells remain healthy. But if you say, "No, I am too old," naturally the blood circulation recedes. If the rains don't come, there is drought and famine, and if you don't do yoga—if you don't irrigate the body—then when you get drought or famine in the body as incurable diseases, you just accept them and prepare to die.

Why should you allow the drought to come when you can irrigate the body? If you could not irrigate it at all, it would be a different matter. But when it is possible to irrigate, you should surely do so. Not to do so allows the offensive forces to increase and the defensive forces to decrease. Disease is an offensive force; inner-energy is a defensive force. As we grow older the defensive strength gets less and the offensive strength increases. That is how diseases enter into our system. A body which carries out yogic practice is like a fort which keeps up its defensive strength so that the offensive strength in the form of diseases will not enter into it through the skin. Which do you prefer? Yoga helps to maintain the defensive strength at an optimum level, and that is what is known as health.

I have been doing yoga for over 50 years and have taught many thousands of students in the five continents of this globe. Sadly, there are teachers of yoga who know very little and claim to teach. The problem comes not from the art of yoga, but from the inexperience of the teachers and also from the impatience of the pupils. If a person who cannot stand tries to walk, he will break his legs, and so it is with yoga. In Western countries particularly, people want above all to do *Padmasana*, the Lotus Pose. They say, "I think I can do it!" Unfortunately, the thinking is in the head, but the doing is in the knee! If you do not understand the intelligence of the knee and you force it to follow your brain, then the knee will break. But if you understand the stiffness as well as the mobility of the knee, and go step by step to remove the stiffness and increase the range of mobility, then there is no danger at all. If there are accidents in yoga, it is not the fault of yoga, but of the aggressiveness of the pupil who does it.

So you can all do yoga. The Queen of Belgium started doing Head Balance at the age of 86. Nothing happened to her. I hope there will be no confusion about what I am saying. You can do it, but do it judiciously, knowing your capacity. If you try to imitate me, naturally you will suffer, because I have been doing it for a century. You have to wait to reach that level. Yoga cannot be rushed.

Excerpted from *The Tree of Yoga*, by B.K.S. Iyengar, pp. 31-34, 1988. B.K.S. Iyengar. Reprinted by arrangement with Shambhala Publications, Inc.

Eleven

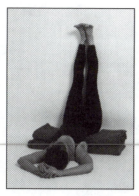

Restful Inversions: The Elixir of Life

I started yoga during a sad period, because I had lost my husband and I was very run down. With yoga I could survive. . . . It is such a shock when someone near you dies. Yoga helped me. I didn't know it would help, because I did it like I did tennis or a game—it was fun for me. But it went much deeper than I could understand at that point. I saw this later on. . . . A new life came into my body. In nature the flowers blossom in the spring and then again in the autumn. I felt this.

—VANDA SCARAVELLI, ADAPTED FROM AN INTERVIEW BY ESTHER MYERS AND KIM ECHLIN, *YOGA JOURNAL*, MAY/JUNE 1996

Legs-Up-the-Wall Pose

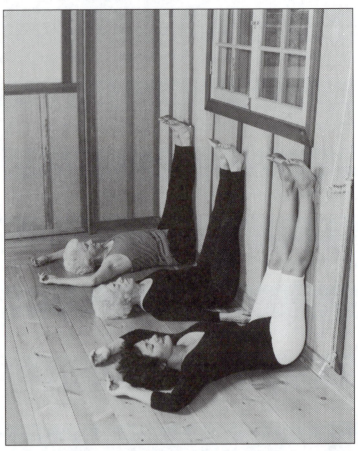

I recommend this restorative pose to everyone. It is sheer bliss!

The benefits of Legs-Up-the-Wall Pose confirm the wisdom in the old-fashioned phrase, "Put your legs up." Few things are easier and more refreshing after standing upright all day than lying on your back and elevating your legs on a wall.

Relaxing with your legs up on a wall is a safe and soothing way to get used to inverting your body. I have taught this pose to many people who had difficulty getting down to the floor and scooting their body close enough to the wall. If lying close to a wall is truly not feasible for you, a friend or companion can bring the "wall" to you in the form of a tall, straight-backed, sturdy chair, and you can elevate your legs against its back. If even getting down on the floor is not practical for you, consider placing your bed beside a bare wall. Then you can relax with your legs up the wall while you're lying in bed.

How to Practice Legs-Up-the-Wall Pose

1. Sit on the floor beside a wall, knees bent, with one shoulder and hip touching the wall.
2. Now roll your weight onto your opposite elbow and shoulder and swing around to bring your legs up the wall so that you end up lying on your back. Many beginners inadvertently move too far away from the wall when they first try this, so you may need to wriggle your bottom closer to the wall. Most people feel more comfortable with their bottom a few inches away from the wall, especially if their legs are quite stiff. Position yourself so that your back and your legs feel relaxed. At my yoga center, students learn this pose within reach of the wall ropes and pull on the ropes to get close to the wall.
3. Be sure your pelvis is relaxing on the floor and that your back feels comfortable. If you are uncomfortable lying with your bottom close to the wall, scoot back a few inches until your body feels more relaxed, or try bending your knees a bit to ease the backs of your legs.

As in other lying down positions, it is important that your head and neck feel comfortable. Notice if your head tilts back, and your chin is higher than your forehead. If so, place a firm, folded blanket under your head and neck so that your forehead is slightly higher than your chin. An eyebag or other cover over your eyes will deepen the feeling of relaxation.

Stay in the pose about five minutes at first, then gradually increase the time. Let your mind follow the soft rise and fall of your breath. Allow your breathing to slow down and relax, as described in the section on breathing and the heart in chapter 9. When you are ready to come out of the pose, remove the cover from your eyes and lie still for a few more breaths with your eyes open. Then bend your knees toward your chest, turn to your side and with the help of your arms uncurl slowly back to a sitting position or to Child's Pose.

You can also conveniently follow Legs-Up-the-Wall Pose with a few minutes of active stretching before you sit up. Stretch your inner thighs by slowly widening the legs, or do a lying-down variation of the Bound-Angle Pose by bending your knees and bringing the soles of your feet together. Or, you can cross your ankles, allowing the wall to support your feet. Some people feel more comfortable with a folded blanket under their bottom.

If you practiced Legs-Up-the-Wall at the beginning of your yoga practice, you can follow it with the invigorating Downward-Facing Dog Pose, since you are already kneeling on the floor. If done at the end of your practice, follow with Deep Relaxation Pose (chapter 12) or other relaxing positions.

In the 20 years that I have taught people of all ages and conditions, I have not come across anyone who did not feel the benefits from this simple inverted pose. People who were bedridden, sometimes incontinent, found the pose a great relief, especially when their legs and feet were swollen from retaining water. For people who spend long periods in bed or in a wheelchair, this pose is even more important. Lying in bed with the soles of the feet together, the feet elevated on a pile of extra large firm pillows or a stack of firm, neatly folded blankets, provides a relief similar to Legs-Up-the Wall Pose.

Cautions: People with heart problems, neck problems, eye pressure, retinal problems or hiatal hernia should use caution with all inverted poses. However, Legs-Up-the-Wall Pose is recommended for people with mild hypertension because it can help normalize blood pressure. Such people should gradually increase the length of time spent in the pose until they are spending at least 15 minutes a day.

Beginning yoga students with high blood pressure, heart problems or other medical considerations are advised to help the body become accustomed to inverting by regularly lying down with the legs resting on the seat of a chair, or practicing in bed with a stack of firm pillows or folded blankets. For some, this position will be appropriate for several weeks, then they may graduate to relaxing with the legs up on the wall.

These simple inverted positions are especially beneficial for people who stand for long periods of time, those whose legs and feet swell easily, or anyone with varicose veins.

Supported Legs-Up-the-Wall Pose (Viparita Karani)

In Sanskrit, *Viparita* means "inverted." *Karani* refers to a particular type of practice. This pose is also known as a variation of Supported Shoulderstand.

Mental clarity comes
from a clean colon
and a straight spine.
—*Hindu proverb*

Viparita Karani is a gentle, supported Legs-Up-the-Wall inverted pose that can be practiced by almost everyone. It is a safe, non-threatening position that most people can hold long enough for gravity to return the blood from the extremities to the vital organs. This pose can generally be practiced by people who are too weak or debilitated for other inversions. Viparita Karani is especially valuable during times of fatigue, low energy, illness and stress.

The way this restful, restorative yoga posture gently inverts the body without effort, it is almost physiologically impossible not to relax deeply. The "work" lies in learning how best to arrange your body—but once the body is in the right position, your job is to let go of all effort and just enjoy the feeling of relaxing.

Viparita Karani is considered the most healing of the yoga restorative poses. When we turn upside down, gravity helps the venous blood—which otherwise tends to pool in the legs—to return easily to the heart. In people whose heart rates are elevated because they have not been receiving an ample supply of blood, Viparita Karani reduces the heart rate by improving the blood flow into the chest. In this gentle supported inversion, as in other more active inverted postures, the weight of the blood in the feet, legs and abdomen stimulates blood pressure receptors in the neck and chest to reduce the constriction of the arteries throughout the body. This reduces blood pressure.

Part of the soothing effect derived from Viparita Karani is due to the angle of the torso. Note in the photo how the stack of blankets positioned under the pelvis brings the torso into a gentle supported backbend, while the legs are supported by the wall. As we lie in the pose, we can imagine that its shape creates an internal waterfall, as the fluid in the legs cascades down to the abdomen and spills over into the chest, toward the heart. The blood seems to cascade like a gentle waterfall toward the heart in a smooth, controlled flow. This waterfall effect creates a peaceful, soothing sensation.

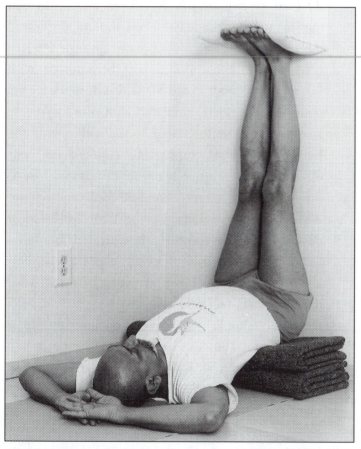

A sandbag placed on the feet by a helper deepens the feeling of relaxation in the Viparita Karani pose.

How to Practice Viparita Karani

1. Have available three firm blankets, or yoga bolsters or other firm cushions. If you use blankets or sofa

cushions, they must provide a firm, level support. The width of the blanket depends somewhat on your height and flexibility. For most people, the edge of the blanket can be placed at the waist. This placement allows the back to curve in such a way that the lower lumbar spine is protected. Note that the blankets support the buttocks in such a way that the ribcage is spread. The chest should appear and feel very open, so that the breath can flow freely.

2. It is generally helpful to first be familiar with Legs-Up-the-Wall Pose. Sit with your side to the wall, your folded blankets within easy reach. Keeping your bottom close to the wall, swing the legs up the wall, supporting yourself on your elbow and forearms. When your bottom is close to the wall, relax your arms and lie back on the floor. As described in Legs-Up-the-Wall Pose, most people feel more comfortable with their bottom a few inches away from the wall, especially if their legs are quite stiff. Position yourself so that your back and legs feel relaxed.

3. Beginners should wait to proceed until this feels comfortable. The next step is to place one or two blankets under your bottom, with your lower back supported. When this feels comfortable, a third blanket or fourth blanket can be added to open the chest even more. Experiment with the height of your blankets or bolster so that their support feels just right for your body—not too high or too low. If your neck or shoulders are uncomfortable, experiment with a small folded towel under the head or shoulders. The neck must feel comfort-able—without any tightness or pinching at the

nape. If blood flow to the head is obstructed, the brain cannot relax.

4. Close your eyes and cover them with a soft folded cloth or eyebag. Observe the rise and fall of your breath. Allow your heart and chest area to relax and open. Stay in the position a minimum of 5 minutes —10 to 15 minutes is preferable. You may find yourself falling asleep.

5. When you are ready to come out, bend your knees and slide your body away from the wall. Lie on the floor for a few more breaths before you turn to your side and slowly sit up.

Viparita Karani refreshes the heart and lungs, works to restore depleted energy and rebuild energy reserves. It is deeply relaxing during times of stress and tension and has a beneficial effect on the immune system. As we stay in the pose, the agitation and fatigue that accompany stress fade away.

Supported Shoulderstand (Salamba Sarvangasana)

The Shoulderstand, known as the queen or mother of the yoga postures, is one of the greatest gifts the ancient yogis have given us. (See photos in the menopause section, chapter 6, pages 128-129, and on pages 234-235 in this chapter.) This posture brings health, happiness and harmony to the mind and body. It restores our energy reserves and brings a feeling of quiet and lightness. It is practically a panacea for most ills of the body, considering the circulatory, respiratory, eliminative and endocrine benefits. According to B.K.S. Iyengar, the Shoulderstand helps to regulate metabolism by stimulating the thyroid and parathyroid glands at the base of the throat, a region that is gently compressed during Shoulderstand. Because this pose allows fluid to drain naturally from the lungs and it effectively expands the chest, Shoulderstand is excellent for people suffering from respiratory problems.

The inversion of the body in Shoulderstand profoundly affects the circulatory system. When we are in a standing position, blood must be pumped against the force of gravity back to the heart from the lower extremities. In Shoulderstand, blood flows to the heart effortlessly, without taxing the heart or constricting the arteries. It is this boost to the circulatory system that gives the Shoulderstand its fatigue-relieving properties.

Please read the instructions for the Shoulderstand all the way through several times before proceeding. While you can learn how to practice this pose on your own from a book or tape, these tools are even more valuable as a way of reinforcing what you learn in class. Especially when it comes to the safe practice of inverted poses, I cannot emphasize too strongly that the guidance of an instructor is invaluable for learning these healing, rejuvenating poses. (See also Cautions at the end of this chapter.)

How to Practice Supported Shoulderstand at the Wall

The support of a wall or a chair placed at the sacrum helps you to straighten your back, open your chest, relax and stay in the pose longer. It is advisable to have a teacher assist you with placing the chair the first few times you practice this way. I suggest that you be familiar with Shoulderstand at the Wall before practicing with a chair.

In Shoulderstand, the back of your head is on the floor, with the shoulders evenly placed about an inch from the edge of the blanket. The purpose of elevating the shoulders on a stack of blankets is to protect the neck. Keep your neck soft and relaxed. In Shoulderstand the cervical vertebrae, the smallest and weakest of the spinal bones, are in a most vulnerable position. The raised platform of folded blankets is used to lift the neck away from the floor. The tops of your shoulders come close to the edge of the blanket, the back of your head touches the floor and the neck retains its normal curve.

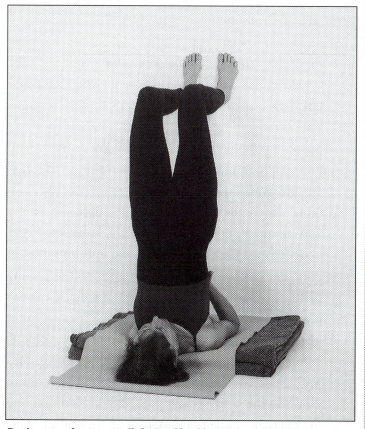

Putting your feet on a wall during Shoulderstand can help you straighten your back and gradually learn to balance in this pose.

The bones of the neck should not press into the floor. To avoid injury, do not turn your head in Shoulderstand. Keep your chin in line with your chest.

Prepare a set of three to five folded blankets, with the folded edges neatly together. In general, the height of the blanket should be two to three inches, and wide enough to support your shoulders and elbows. Shoulderstand may seem easier without having to fold all those blankets, but there is a tendency for the neck to feel strain and pressure from the unaccustomed weight of the body. The height of the blankets varies according to the length and flexibility of your neck. Your teacher can help you to determine the right number of blankets to use.

1. Place the firm, folded blankets near a wall, with the folded edges away from the wall. The exact distance away from the wall depends on the length of your torso.
2. Sit on the blankets beside a wall, knees bent, with one shoulder and hip touching the wall, as in Legs-Up-the-Wall Pose.
3. Now shift your weight onto your opposite elbow and shoulder and swivel your trunk around to bring your legs up the wall, so that you end up lying on your back, your shoulders well supported by the blankets, the back of your neck and head off the blankets.
4. Many beginners inadvertently slip off the blankets when they first try this pose. As in Legs-Up-the-Wall Pose, you may need to wriggle your bottom closer to the wall, so that your shoulders remain on the blankets while your legs are up the wall. If your shoulders fall off the blankets when your bottom is

close to the wall, try placing the blankets a little farther away from the wall, to accommodate the length of your torso.

5. Bend your knees, press the soles of the feet against the wall, raise your hips and chest off the floor until your back feels straight. Firmly support your back with both hands, bringing your elbows closer together. Make sure your shoulders have remained on the blankets and the back of your head on the floor. The neck should feel comfortable without pressure or pain. Do not turn your neck once you are in this position. If you feel comfortable, stay for several minutes, gradually increasing your stay in the pose. When you are ready to come down, place your hands back on the floor, bend your knees, and gently lower your back and bottom to the floor.

You can relax with your legs up on the wall a few more minutes by sliding back off the blankets till your shoulders touch the floor. When you feel ready to sit up, bend your knees, turn to your side and slowly sit up. Or you can remain lying down and follow this pose with some gentle floor twists.

Shoulderstand and Plow Pose with Chairs

Study the photos on the following page carefully and note the positioning of the props. If you are new in class, it is important to have an opportunity to see your teacher or another student demonstrate the pose before you attempt it. Again, your teacher can help you determine the number of blankets that works best for you. In the beginning, you may need the help of a teacher to position

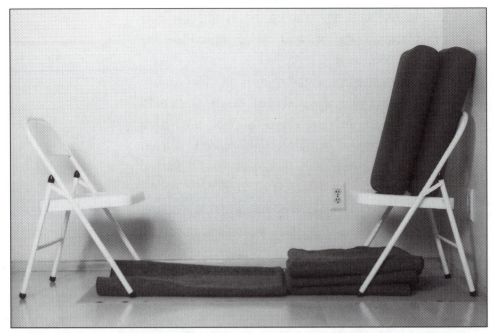

A set-up of two chairs, blankets and bolsters as shown can help you safely practice Shoulderstand and Plow Pose.

the chairs. Later, you can use the chairs independently. For added security, place the back of the chair against a wall for Shoulderstand. Two bolsters can be placed on the seat of the chair, as illustrated, to further increase your stability, openness and the length of time you remain in the pose.

1. Position the neatly folded blankets so that when you lie down, your shoulders are still on the blankets. Your bottom should be near the front edge of the chair and your lower legs should rest on the seat. You should be close enough to the chair to grasp its front legs.

2. Place a second chair far enough behind you so that when you lower your legs, your feet will rest on the seat of the chair.

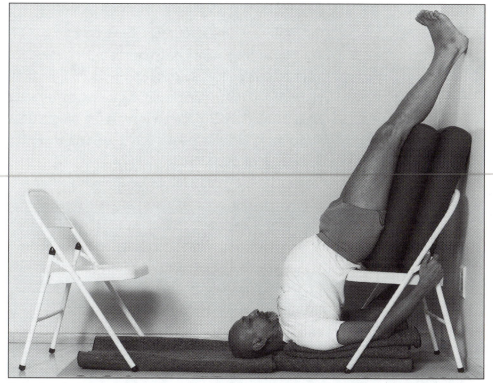

Reversing gravity reverses the aging process. Supporting the hips and back of legs makes this pose secure and relaxing.

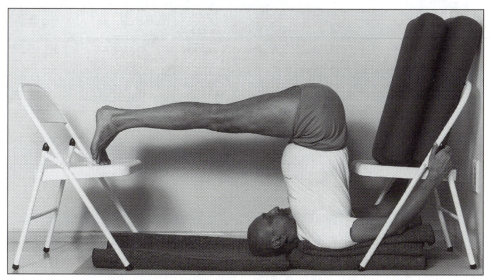

Notice the vertical position of the back and 90-degree angle formed by the legs.

3. Bend your legs and place your feet on the edge of the chair seat. Press your feet into the chair, and lift your torso till you are on your shoulders. Interlace your fingers and stretch your arms toward the front chair. If your arms don't touch the floor with your fingers interlaced, place your arms flat on the floor and press into the floor with your palms. Relax your neck, throat and face.

4. When you feel ready to proceed, place your hands firmly on your back, as close to your shoulders as possible. Bring your elbows in toward each other, in line with your shoulders, and open your chest.

5. When you feel stable and secure here, exhale and lift one leg up to the ceiling. On the next exhalation, lift the other leg. Hold for a few breaths, straightening your back as much as possible.

6. Exhale and lower one leg at a time onto the chair behind you. When your feet are secure on the chair, release your hands off your back and reach for the legs of the chair. Move the chair toward you until it touches your back.

7. With your arms inside the legs of the chair, hold the back legs of the chair, near the seat as illustrated. When you feel ready to proceed, lift one leg at a time to the ceiling, pulling the chair toward you and firmly grasping the back legs. Stretch up through your legs and feet. With practice, you will come higher up on your shoulders and your body will be straighter. As you feel more comfortable, increase the length of time in this position.

8. Lower your feet one at a time to the chair, until the tips of your toes touch the chair seat. Stretch your bottom up toward the ceiling, lengthening your

spine. Hold the position about half a minute, gradually increasing your time in the pose.

9. There are several ways you can come out of the pose. With your feet on the chair, push the chair at your back away from you (or to the side if it is braced against a wall). Place your hands on the floor behind your back and lower your back slowly down, keeping your head on the floor. Bend your knees and place your feet on the floor. Slide back off the blanket until your shoulders are completely on the floor. Relax in this lying down position for a few more minutes.

Cautions: As discussed in chapter 2, inverted positions, whether done with special equipment or on your own, are only as safe as people learn to practice them. While simple inversions such as Legs-Up-the-Wall Pose and Viparita Karani can generally be learned on your own, other inverted poses should ideally be learned under the guidance of an experienced teacher.

People with the following conditions should not practice inversions without the supervision of a physician or an experienced yoga teacher: high blood pressure; glaucoma or detached retina; hiatal hernia; heart problems or stroke; epilepsy, seizures, or other brain disorders; temporary conditions such as acute infections of the ear, throat or sinuses; obesity; conditions requiring aspirin therapy; chronic neck problems, whiplash or osteoporosis. People with neck injuries or conditions such as cervical spondylosis must take care to avoid yoga poses that involve weight-bearing directly on the spine, as in Headstand and Shoulderstand.

Indra Devi:
Yoga Defies Aging

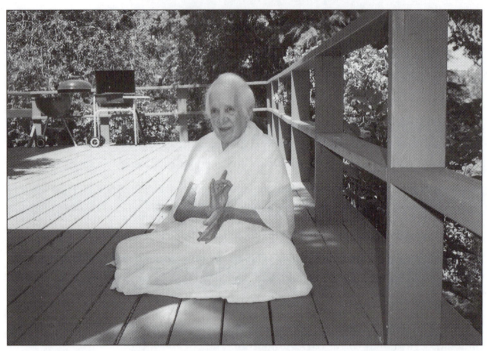

Indra Devi at age 94.

After a year of fruitless phone calls, I finally managed to catch up with Indra Devi, one of this century's most renowned and beloved yoga teachers. Born Eugenie Peterson on May 12, 1899, in Riga, Russia, she explains in the introduction to her book, Forever Young, Forever Healthy, *that even as a child she was irresistibly drawn to India. She left Moscow in 1920 to become an actress and dancer, and traveled throughout Europe, where she met J. Krishnamurti. In 1927 she arrived in India. During the first four months of her stay there, she traveled extensively. She met Mahatma Gandhi and other leading spiritual and political figures. After many mishaps and adventures, she unexpectedly became an Indian movie star, and renamed herself Indra Devi.*

She married a Czechoslovakian diplomat and her spiritual aspirations fell by the wayside as her life became one of parties and worldly pleasures. During this period she developed severe health problems, which lasted several years and almost killed her. A remarkable series of events led her to study yoga with T. Krishnamacharya, a highly regarded yogi who also taught T.K.V. Desikachar and B.K.S. Iyengar. In 1939 Indra Devi followed her husband to Shanghai, China, where she opened her first yoga school.

Returning to India in the mid-1940s, she retreated to the Himalayas, where she wrote the first of a series of bestselling yoga books that were eventually translated into 10 languages. From then on she has lectured on yoga all over the world. In the late 1940s, when people were still confusing yoga with yogurt, she established a yoga school in Hollywood, California, where her students included Gloria Swanson and Olivia de Haviland.

On the day of my interview with Indra Devi, I arrived half an hour early. She was still in her nightgown and slippers, her wild white hair uncombed.

"Oh," she laughed, eyes twinkling and looking every bit like some mischievous, impish child clad in a wise old woman's body, "usually people are late!" The fact that she did not dash into the bathroom to dress made me feel like a close friend or member of the family. "Well," I thought, "the First Lady of Yoga has nothing to hide and doesn't give a hoot about first impressions." I also noted with great relief that she still painted her nails pink—laying to rest my fears that one must renounce frivolous feminine rituals in order to tread the spiritual path. I expected to have to wait until Indra Devi dressed and finished her breakfast, but she motioned for me to sit at the table and get started. Here is an excerpt of what Indra Devi had to say:

I know you're writing a book of yoga for people who are aging. Just a few days ago I was interviewed for the newspaper, the radio and the television, all at the same time. The radio man asked, "How does it feel—aging?" I said, I don't know how it feels. Ask someone who's aging. I don't know anything about aging.

People don't have to wait to do yoga until they're aging. But what can you do? Usually that's how people are. Not until something happens to their body—then they start thinking about it. People allow their body to become old, stiff, fat or whatever by doing everything wrong. From exercising, to eating, to thinking.

If you think yourself old, you will become old. Youth comes from inside. Of course, for people over 80 who are already aging, yoga can do a lot of things for reversing the aging process. They can start with yoga exercises that everybody can do. But just doing only the physical part of yoga is not enough. You have to do things that affect your mind. You must make your mind like an arrow when you want to do something, and not be distracted.

Whatever is in the physical world can be translated into the spiritual world. In the physical world, if you want to be a musician, like a pianist, what do you have to do? Hours and hours of practicing. The same thing in the spiritual world. You want to achieve something, you have to work, but a different kind of work. The practice of yoga is invaluable. Yoga affects all of our faculties, physical, mental and spiritual.

I start with the physical body, deep relaxation and deep breathing. Deep breathing is an exercise you don't do all the time. You start with five or six deep breaths, filling the entire lungs, starting from the lower part and on upward. But very few people take the time to practice this. Most of our life we use only one-third of our lung capacity, the upper part. Many people don't even know they have a lower part. The lower part of your lungs is not for decoration. You first start with five, six or seven deep breaths. You can practice this in the fresh air two or three times a day. And then gradually more. Sixty deep breaths a day guarantees you to be in good health and good spirits.

I practice every day. Some people say, "Oh, I don't feel the need." What do they mean? You breathe every day. You eat every day. That's why you should continue to practice the yoga exercises. You might not feel the need today, but three years later you will feel the need! You should not practice yoga only when you are in pain or discomfort, then give it up because the pain is gone.

Twelve

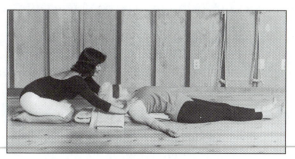

Savasana, Pose of Deep Relaxation

When a member of my extended family died, I did not feel inspired to practice my usual yoga routine. In response to my grief, I decided to practice only restorative poses, and did so almost every day for a year. It was practicing these poses, I believe, that helped me through this extremely painful period. They opened me in a way that allowed me to accept my pain and to recover from the emotional drain and fatigue.

—Judith Lasater, Ph.D., P.T. *Relax & Renew: Restful Yoga for Stressful Times*

In Sanskrit, *Sava*, or *Shava*, means "corpse." In this pose, the body lies on the floor face up and completely relaxed, while the mind is at ease and alert. The eyes are closed, the arms relaxed at the sides, the palms up. The body remains as still and motionless as a corpse.

The influence of this asana on the body and the mind—from relaxation, to surrender, to death, and even after death—is incredible. If you do not want to be a living corpse, then the purpose of life has to be established. If you want to be an active participant in your life and not a parasite, then the dynamic interdependence between life and death has to be recognized, and the two have to meet in directed and concentrated interaction.

In Shavasana, relaxation is the first attempt to surrender, to let go. As the mind follows the flow of the breath, the ripples of the mental lake slowly subside. With continued practice, the senses are gradually withdrawn and become still. Passion, egocentricity, self-importance are, for the moment, put to rest. Rest becomes an important word whose meaning expands with experience. Shavasana, the corpse posture, gives a new understanding of death, of the need for surrender. The body at rest can do its repair work. Sufficient rest allows the body to recuperate from the driving forces of the emotions and the ambitions of the mind. The benefits—physically, mentally, emotionally—are profound. In that state of peace and quiet and inner harmony, one can perceive a vision of the Light that is present in both life and death.

—Swami Sivananda Radha
Hatha Yoga: The Hidden Language

Although *Savasana,* the classic Pose of Deep Relaxation, might seem like the easiest posture to practice, those who delve deeply into the art of yoga realize that it is among the most difficult poses to master.

In Savasana, the body lies still and silent—empty of agitation, mimicking a corpse. The mind is in the present, alert and aware, serene, detached, observing while the body releases deeply and lets go. In this state of conscious relaxation, the body and mind are recharged, refreshed and rejuvenated. This condition of deep rest allows the body and mind to be profoundly quiet and at peace.

Setting aside at least five minutes at the end of your yoga session to consciously relax is healthful for your whole being. To consciously relax removes fatigue from the body, soothes the nerves and brings a feeling of pleasant calmness and happiness. Deep relaxation—which is very different from flopping in front of the television and falling asleep—is healing. Physiologically, such relaxation is characterized by a slower heart rate, metabolism and rate of breathing, lower blood pressure, and slower brain wave patterns.

> The yogic art of relaxation known as Savasana puts down in precise steps how relaxation and recuperation take place. Savasana is a posture that simulates a dead body, and evokes the experience of remaining in a state as in death and of ending the heartaches and shocks that the flesh is heir to. It means relaxation and therefore recuperation. It is not simply lying on one's back with a vacant mind and gazing, nor does it end in snoring. It is the most difficult of yogic asanas to perfect, but it is also the most refreshing and rewarding.
> —B.K.S.Iyengar
> Light on Pranayama

The Art of Conscious Relaxation

Learning to consciously relax takes practice. Choose a warm, quiet place where you will not be disturbed. Have an extra blanket available in cooler weather to cover yourself if needed. Remove contact lenses or glasses.

In this pose the body is placed evenly on the floor. If your head tilts back or feels uncomfortable, place a folded blanket under your head and neck, thick enough to bring your forehead slightly higher than your chin. If your back feels uncomfortable when you straighten your legs, then bend your knees and place a pillow or folded blanket under your knees to help you relax or support your calves on the seat of a chair.

1. Sit on the floor with your legs straight out in front of you. Lean back on your elbows and check that your upper body and legs are in line. If not, adjust the position of your torso or your legs so that your chin, center of your chest, navel and pubic bone extend directly toward a center point between your heels.

2. Lower your back slowly to the floor. Place a blanket under your head as needed. Allow your back to sink toward the floor.

3. Turn the upper arms out, slightly away from the trunk, palms up. Extend the arms out of the shoulders, then allow them to relax. Soften your hands, allowing your fingers to curl naturally.

4. Extend the legs and feet. Allow them to drop toward the floor and fall evenly away from the midline. Soften your toes.

5. Close your eyes. Relax your lips and tongue. Let your lower jaw be loose, your lips barely touching, your tongue passive. Allow your mouth to feel as if you are about to smile. Feel your face muscles soften and relax. Let your eyes sink deep in their sockets. Allow your body to release and sink toward the floor.

6. As you lie still, let your mind follow your breath. Quietly observe the peaceful in-and-out flow of your inhalation and exhalation. Listen to the beat of your own heart. Each time your mind starts to wander into the past or future, bring your awareness back to the breath.

Stay lying still for about five or 10 minutes, or longer.

Let go of the past—become "dead" to the old and prepare the way for something new.

Deep relaxation is also considered a preparation for conscious death. Letting go of the fears and morbid misunderstandings associated with the death of the physical body may help prepare us for the mysterious transition from life to death.

Regular practice of deep relaxation will leave you feeling refreshed, rejuvenated and optimistic.

Note again that it is of utmost importance that your head and back position are comfortable. Check that the height under your head is thick enough so that your forehead is slightly higher than your chin. Your head should not drop back and pinch your neck. Experiment with the thickness of the blanket under your head until it feels right. Keep your knees bent if your back feels more comfortable in this position.

As described in chapter 3, an eyebag over your eyes will help you relax. An eye covering helps quiet the mind by creating darkness and removing visual stimuli, by relaxing the muscles around your eyes and by calming the involuntary movements of your eyes.

Savasana Variation

Relax deeply by lying evenly on two or three blankets folded lengthwise under the lower back, chest and head, with an extra blanket placed under the head so that the forehead does not drop back. Supporting the length of your spine and back of the head with firmly folded blankets opens the chest, allowing the breath to flow freely—especially beneficial to people with heart and respiratory problems. For those who suffer from depression and low energy, a relaxing position that opens the chest can be a lifesaver.

Refer back to chapters 3, 6 and 10 to review the use of eyebags, bolsters and folded blankets for deep relaxation.

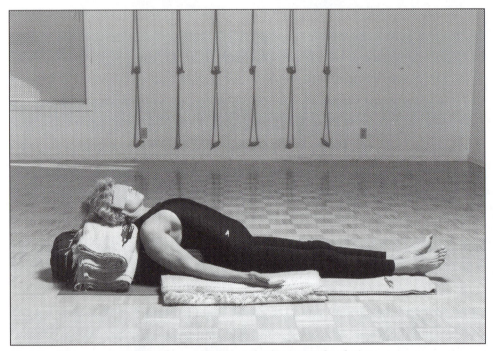

Find the right amount of support for your body to make this pose truly relaxing.

Diana Clifton:
Letting Go of Pain, Learning to Relax

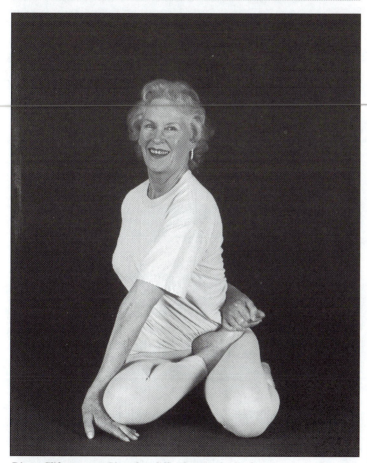

Diana Clifton at age 73 makes difficult poses look easy.

To be in a class with Diana is to experience the soul of yoga. Her extraordinary knowledge of poses and gentle, deeply penetrating manner open fresh lines of perception, depth and self-inquiry. She reminds one of the river in Siddhartha*—sharing its secrets endlessly with those who hear, and yet in the ordinary passage of its flow, simply carrying many across from one side to the other.*

—Anonymous Student

Diana Clifton, an inspiring teacher who lives in England, did not begin practicing yoga or become health- and nutrition-conscious until she was in her 40s, at which time she says she was someone who was in poor health with anemia, constipation, nervousness and fatigue.

Three decades later, she makes difficult postures look effortless, reminding students half her age that yoga postures are natural—young children can do most of them with ease! Like many older people, Diana experienced the loss of a spouse. We discussed many aspects of yoga and life—including aging, death and depression. Diana described the year she spent nursing her sick husband and the overwhelming grief and exhaustion she felt when he died.

We all have to face death. I think you have to die while you're still alive. That means renouncing everything before your death—goods, wealth, friends, relations, loved ones. Mind you, you can't take anything with you when you die. Older students know that. This realization might bring them to a point of silence. You see, I believe that death is such a natural thing. It's only the death of the body. We are not the body. So, strictly speaking, we don't die anyway. It's only the physical that goes—that includes our possessions, of course. But after all, you close your eyes and they're gone. So, it's our senses we hold on to most.

There is great duality in life. One is joy—one is pain. We all embrace joy, but we do not embrace pain. And why is that? Maybe we could look at our pain for a little while and become detached from it. It's hard to do. A lot of the pain is stress. Yoga can teach you how to let go, how to relax.

Older people starting yoga can lie flat on their backs, for a start. A support under their neck and head, and a yoga bolster or folded blankets under the back to open the chest, will help them to breathe and relax. Ask students to watch their breath and look at their own thoughts. If someone comes to yoga, something inside them has prompted them. It may not be merely because of their suffering, physically. It may be more than that. It may be because they haven't found any comfort in their religion. As it is now, a lot of people don't find comfort in religion. And if they can discover what's inside themselves, so that they don't need a religion, so that they don't need love from another, because the love is within them; if they can discover the love within themselves, and if you, as a teacher, have got love within yourself—at a certain point, maybe, once the ego has dropped—there is serenity. Once the ego has dropped, they can relax. Teach them how to relax lying on their back in Savasana. A short session of gentle stretching first will make it easier for them to relax.

For depression, you have to open the chest. Because if the chest is concave, they won't get over their depression. So they must open the chest by lying on the floor, placing bolsters or folded blankets under the chest. And then have them watch their breathing.

One thing you can tell them while they're lying in Savasana is to keep the inhalation and exhalation the same length. So, while they're working on their breathing they can think about this. It not only helps the student to concentrate, but it's also better, from the breathing point of view, if they exhale completely. Say they count to 10 on the exhalation—then they should count to 10 on the inhalation. If one is longer than the other, they have to shorten the long one, not to try to overdo it. And also—if they can, pause at the end of the exhalation, because often there's a lot of air still there and, if they pause, that's the deepest point in relaxation. You tell them about this way of breathing, but also explain not to do it if it's a strain. You help them understand that the breathing is cleansing.

Thirteen

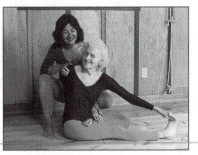

Tips on Teaching and Hints for Home Practice

As your body becomes more flexible, you become more flexible in how you interact in your life and more possibilities open up. People become more aware that they can do more things as a result of establishing strength and then becoming more flexible. When you start to do things that you never did as a child, as I have found in my 50s and 60s, it's just incredible. You feel that life can just keep opening up for you, instead of closing down.

—TONI MONTEZ, YOGA TEACHER

Older students come to yoga with various levels of abilities and medical histories. Some athletic 60-year-olds are soon practicing

Handstands at the wall. Others gain confidence by beginning with simpler poses done lying on the floor. Both teacher and student need to remember that, "Expectations determine outcome." With rare exceptions, I expect students of all ages to practice the vital weight-bearing standing postures that safely stretch and strengthen the whole body. For older beginners, it helps to introduce the poses at a slower pace and encourage students with balance or other problems to make intelligent use of walls, wall ropes, chairs and other props.

Don't treat me like an old lady!
—78-year-old student to her teacher

As I stated in the introduction, older people start yoga for most of the same reasons as other people. They want to feel better, have more energy, improve their posture, strength and flexibility. However, many older students also come to yoga when everyday activities become more and more difficult for them. They hope the practice of yoga will help them remain mobile and return them to their normal ability to function, instead of becoming increasingly incapacitated, and in some cases, facing the very real possibility of spending the last period of their lives having to depend on other people.

The Three Gifts of a Yoga Program for Seniors

1. Yoga improves posture and breathing, thereby improving the health of all the systems of the body.
2. Yoga restores and maintains normal mobility and a healthy range of motion in order to function well in daily life.
3. Yoga helps us to grow and expand psychologically and spiritually. Yoga offers a foundation for conscious living, conscious aging and conscious dying.

The yoga practices presented here are specifically geared to people who need to start exercising gradually. Older beginners who leap enthusiastically into Full Arm Balance during their first class can refer to the more general yoga books listed in the Resources section as their guides.

Guidelines for Teachers of Older Beginners

Many older people have parts of their bodies that have become virtually immobilized. Over time their longstanding physical problems have become magnified. Often these students accept these limitations as an inevitable part of aging and have withdrawn their awareness from their trouble spots, such as a shoulder, knee, foot or hand. It's almost as if that part of the body no longer belongs to them. As they practice the yoga postures, their awareness and sensitivity return. At the same time as this can bring an awakening and new sense of aliveness, it can also increase these students' perception of their other physical problems. Some students then blame them on doing yoga.

The main adjustment for teachers of older beginners is to work at a slower pace. Older people need to conserve their energy. A slower pace allows them to get deeply in touch with what is happening to their bodies during the postures.

Some of the most common physical problems of older students are high blood pressure, osteoporosis and arthritis. A teacher must be aware of how to adapt a student's yoga program to each condition.

- **For beginners with high blood pressure, practicing inverted poses such as Headstand or Shoulderstand**

are not recommended. However, as these students progress, gentle inversions should become a regular part of their practice. Of course, students with hypertension should be encouraged to work in a more relaxed way, to minimize stress and tension.

- **Students with osteoporosis should be extra aware in yoga poses.** Any pose that might place stress on a brittle bone should be practiced very carefully.
- **Arthritic students also need a lot of encouragement**. Although it is essential for them to continue moving the arthritic region, the pain such motion causes induces many students to immobilize the area. They have to be coaxed, bit by bit, to bring mobility back. Often the role of the yoga teacher is to help gently awaken the areas of the body that the older student has deemed frozen or hopeless.

Look at what your people need.
—B.K.S. Iyengar to teachers

A teacher must also be sensitive to the energy level and emotional condition of older students. As I look around at my group of seniors, I am aware that while many of them are having the time of their lives, others are going through difficult periods in their lives. Several are primary caretakers for a dependent spouse, other family member or friend. For them, yoga class may be one of the rare moments that they do something for themselves. For others, yoga class is the social highlight of their week. Often someone in the class is grieving and has little energy. This student may also be on medication for depression. The class atmosphere should be both physically and spiritually uplifting so it doesn't add any additional stress to a student's psyche. A well-rounded class includes invigorating poses to stretch, strengthen and revitalize, and restorative poses to relax and let go.

Ten Important Tips for Teaching Older Students

1. Remember to speak loudly and clearly. Many older people are hard of hearing. Make a point to stand near students who have difficulty hearing. If a student does not respond to directions, it may well be because he or she cannot hear you or, in some cases, clearly see you. You may need to stand directly in front of a student, demonstrating while repeating directions louder and clearer. Instructions must be easy to follow. Most of the time they are better understood when they are visual.

2. Take time to demonstrate what happens when a pose is done with healthy alignment; but, on the other hand, be open to allowing students to learn and explore the poses in their own way as long as they don't hurt themselves. Older students may resist and question more than younger ones, especially, perhaps, if you, the teacher, are much younger.

3. Emphasize the benefits of each posture repeatedly, to motivate students to practice and to help them remember the poses. Share the following points:

   • Breathing reflects and affects our selves and our lives. Learning to breathe more deeply and evenly through the nose increases ventilation and reduces stress on the heart.

   • Asanas release energy in the nervous system and stimulate glands. Most of us are energized by yoga and feel increased vitality.

4. Be playful and creative and make sure your students spend time laughing, relaxing, letting go and having fun.

Old people don't need a younger person telling them what to do.

—Advice from a seasoned teacher

5. Be ever on the alert that you do not impose your own myths about aging on your students. It continues to be a revelation for me as a teacher to witness the extent of the progress made by my older students who practice. There may be long periods of time when students, afraid of losing their balance, do standing poses in ways that do not look right. Outwardly, you see little progress. But if you keep demonstrating, directing and encouraging, one day you will be amazed, as I have been, to see almost everyone in the class suddenly grasp what you've been saying all along.

6. A group dynamic is at work in all classes, but it may be even more noticeable in older groups. The octogenarian who comes to class for the first time and sees people practicing yoga in chairs will assume that this is what is expected and act accordingly. Conversely, the more that older people see their peers practicing more challenging poses, the more they will expect of themselves.

7. Create an atmosphere where students feel comfortable to explore the poses at their own pace. Keep in mind that as people grow older, they very often feel unstable and lose their balance. Remember that if your ability to stand and walk becomes increasingly unsure, the rest of life feels less and less secure. Yoga can help seniors regain confidence. The standing poses re-establish the body's connection to the earth. Students develop a sense of rootedness, stability and balance. Standing on one's own two feet is not generally emphasized in other forms of exercise, yet is invaluable to older people.

8. Always do some type of inversion poses, and gradually encourage students to hold them for longer periods. Inversions counteract the aging process by reversing the gravitational pull on the internal organs and improving the venous return to the heart.

9. Relaxation is often difficult for older people. If you have a class of older adults with many physical problems, which as a group is not very strong or limber, it is generally advisable to begin with simpler lying-down poses and work up to standing postures. Some students may experience discomfort lying down and complain about the hardness of the floor. Check their head and neck position to see that the arch at the back of the neck is not extreme—that the head is not tilted back with the forehead lower than the chin. Hyperextension of the back of the neck can restrict the blood supply to the brain. Place pillows, books (or whatever height-increasing prop is available) under the head, and pillows or folded blankets under the thighs if the lower back does not relax into the floor.

10. While as a society our view of aging is changing by leaps and bounds, the myth that older people are still expected to go downhill will not disappear overnight. Bear in mind that many older people feel increasingly helpless, that they are losing control over what happens to them. As they develop and progress through yoga, their confidence returns when they find the downward spiral can be reversed.

Hints for Getting Down to and Up from the Floor

Few experiences are as demoralizing for older people than falling and being unable to get back up off the floor. If this happens while they are home alone, it can mean waiting many hours until someone comes to help them.

The main concern of many of my older students during their first yoga class is how to get up from and down to the floor. New students often tell me, "I'll just sit in a chair instead of going on the floor." For these people, regaining confidence in moving to and from the floor is the most important part of their first lesson. I assure them that it will get easier with practice. Experienced students are generally sympathetic and give newcomers suggestions and encouragement.

Students unsure about getting up from the floor will find it helpful to lower themselves to the floor, and raise themselves back up, holding onto a sturdy chair braced securely against a wall. Be sure to position the chair so that it will not slip or collapse. A folded blanket on top of a sticky mat on the floor near the seat makes kneeling less painful.

Each student is unique, and safety—avoiding injury—is always my first concern when assessing the strength, flexibility and coordination of someone new. I may stand nearby to make sure the student does not fall, but generally I offer minimal assistance. It has been my experience that the majority of people who come to class unassisted can relearn to get up and down from the floor with ease and confidence.

If I see a student struggling to get up, I suggest, "Try turning to your other side," or "See which side, which

> One day I found myself looking around for something to get hold of to help me get up. Here's what I found to avoid that: From a kneeling position I raised my right knee, put my right hand on it, and with the help of a push from the floor with the left hand, I was up without trouble. Maybe I've invented an exercise. Anyhow, I do it two or three times a day.
> —*Zilpha Main, Reaching Ninety My Way*

arm, which leg, is stronger." It usually does the trick. If the problem is simply that the student is very weak or stiff and just isn't in the habit of getting up and down off the floor, I often just leave that person alone. Aside from providing a chair or other sturdy object, I let these students figure it out for themselves—which is often what they prefer, rather than drawing attention to their dilemma. I might assure struggling students that it doesn't matter if it takes five or 10 minutes to get up and that, as with everything else, this ability improves with practice. My students who first had difficulty hardly think twice about it now.

Remember this Golden Rule about almost any physical activity: Use it or lose it. Suggest that students avoid sitting in chairs whenever possible; sit on the floor the way children do. Urge them to rise from and descend to the floor at least once a day. When the neuromuscular pathways for getting up and down are used regularly, it is easier to recover if, by chance, you should slip and fall.

Practical Hints for Moving to and from the Floor

1. Stand next to a sturdy chair or other piece of furniture near a wall. If balance is very unstable or leg muscles are very weak, try standing in between two chairs or other stable supports on which you can brace or hold. From standing, holding on to the support as needed, step forward and begin to lower your knees to the floor.

2. Kneeling on both knees, lower your bottom toward your heels. In our chair-oriented culture, where

Growing acquaintance with once-foreign cultures, new discoveries about our subliminal depth, and the dawning recognition that each social group reinforces just some human attributes while neglecting or suppressing others have stimulated a worldwide understanding that all of us have great potential for growth. Perhaps no culture has ever possessed as much publicly available knowledge as we do today regarding the transformative capacities of human nature.

—*Michael Murphy,*
The Future of the Body

hips and leg muscles are often very stiff, many older people have difficulty lowering their bottom to their heels. Holding the chair as needed, try sitting to the side of your feet. Use your arms to lower yourself to the floor. To stand back up, reverse this process. Again, be assured that with daily practice your muscles will strengthen and the movement will become easier. I cannot overemphasize the importance of maintaining the ability to get up and down from the floor. Practicing will also make it easier to get up from chairs and other places, such as the toilet, even if the seat is low.

Wall ropes hanging in many yoga centers are extremely useful for people with balance problems and difficulty getting up and down. They can be ordered for home use from the Resources section.

Barbara Uniker:
I Do Not Accept the Stereotype of Old Age

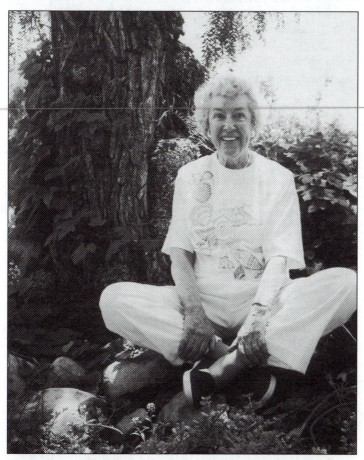

Barbara Uniker's joie de vivre *lights up morning classes at the Ojai Yoga Center.*

About 20 years ago, a friend insisted that I try yoga. It sounded far out, but I agreed, and became rather fascinated. I was surprised to find out that I could even do a Headstand, and other advanced poses. After a year or so, my teacher, Suza Francina, left the area and I discontinued yoga.

As I aged, I became aware that even though I ate nutritiously, did aerobics and was active in community affairs, there was another dimension to be considered. I found myself facing the inevitable diminution of vision, hearing, memory, etc., all of which leads to a loss of confidence and pride. I felt that I was on a downward spiral. It was oh-so-easy to slip into not making an effort, letting things slide, instead of taking steps to do something about situations.

While I was musing about what to do, Suza returned, and I started regular classes with her, knowing that with her both mind and body are stretched. Spiritual values are also part of the picture. Now, the discipline of yoga spurs me on to make more of an effort to learn new poses and hold them longer. The satisfaction derived from success turns the spiral upward and flows into other aspects of living.

Occasionally younger people join our class, and often they are unable to do poses that we practice every class. I enjoy a certain wry satisfaction about that. It encourages me even though I can no longer do a Headstand without help. I know how much yoga has done for me.

It is a sad thought that gravity literally pulls me downward every day of my life. The worst of it settles in my tummy. It cheers me up to know that yoga reverses this pull with its constant stretching upward and inverted poses. While it creates no miracles, it at least gives me an even break.

Another joy from yoga comes from the feeling of relaxation and peace at the end of class. Often I come in tired after early-morning aerobics and various chores and errands. Since the mind as well as the body is cleared in yoga and the spirit is refreshed, it is like starting a new day.

Since concentration is essential to yoga, yoga is an especially good remedy for one of the more difficult problems of aging. For me, yoga classes are an invaluable time for quiet concentration, stretching the mind as well as the body, being spiritually aware and experiencing deep relaxation. The last several years since I have returned to yoga have been especially rewarding ones, telling me that I do not have to accept the stereotype of old age—for I still have much to enjoy in life.

Beatrice Wood:
Age Is Only a Number

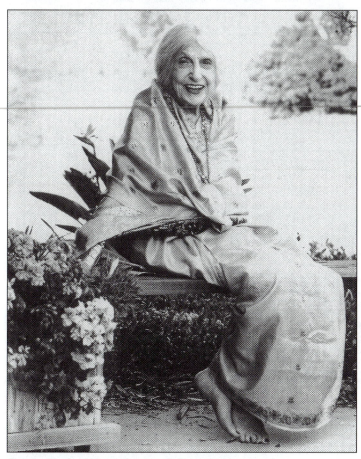

Beatrice Wood at 100—exuberance, daring and joy.

My lifelong friend, Beatrice Wood, a world-renowned potter who took her first ceramics class around age 40, was asked by an interviewer how she felt about aging. Without hesitating she replied: "I have nothing to say. I'm not concerned about it. I may be 100 to you, but to me, I'm 30, so I have no problem."

Over the years, whenever I've eaten with her, I've always noticed that she picks away, like a bird, at her nutritious vegetarian meals, saving room for the most important part—dessert. She reminded me why she does when she turned 103.

"My friends who didn't eat chocolate died a long time ago," she explained. "I don't overindulge. Just a small amount. It makes me feel human."

When I asked her how she felt about dying, she replied: "Isn't death amazing? We all have to die and it's something we can't accept. I have absolutely no concern; when I'm tired I often think I'm practically there. But then, on the other hand, I still want to do quite a few things and I shall be enraged, in heaven, if I can't get them done. I'd go to the great teachers and say, 'Why didn't you let me stay longer?' "

Personally, I think one of her secrets of longevity is that she laughs all the time. "What can one do when one is up against the absurdity of life but laugh," she once told me, adding, "It is curious, but if one smiles, darkness fades."

When I asked about her deep interest in so-called spiritual matters she answered, "I'm very interested in what could be called spirituality, but it doesn't stop me from being very naughty in conversation and even in action. These last few years I've been more or less a nun, but if I fell in love I wouldn't hesitate not to be a nun."

Beatrice meditates every day. She says, "It is in silence that new thoughts come. If we divert the mind with too much distraction, it becomes scrambled like eggs."

Appendix: Understanding the Anatomy of the Spine

~

The average human spine is about 27 inches in length and has four normal curves. The lower back and neck are concave curves; they dip into the body. The tailbone area and rib cage are convex curves—they move out. For optimum health of the spine while stretching, all four curves should be maintained, with no excess (shortening) or rounding in any segment of the spinal column. Any alteration in one curve will affect the curves above or below.

A long, gentle S curve of the spine helps maintain proper spacing between the bones of the spine, the vertebrae. Lengthening the spine to create space between the vertebrae is vital to our health because nerves connected to the organs and structures of the body branch out from the spinal cord between the vertebrae.

The curves of the spine are formed by the different shapes and thicknesses of the individual vertebrae, which are separated and cushioned by disks of cartilage and water. The weight and stress of the body pass through each vertebrae. Between the bones of the spine, disks act like hydraulic "shock absorbers" and allow for movement in all directions. If the curves of the spine become distorted, the spaces between the vertebrae are compressed. This may cause various problems to the disks which are vulnerable to the changing shape of the spine under pressure. The organs and other parts of the body which are stimulated by the corresponding nerves may decline.

By age 30, the blood supply to the disks gradually lessens. In the adult spine, all nourishment to the spine comes from movement. Fluids are drawn in and flushed out of the disks by stretching, lengthening and moving the spine in all directions—forward, backwards, sideways and twisting. If the disks are not nourished, they start to shrink and lose their elasticity, becoming more prone to injury such as herniation and pressure on the sciatic nerve root. When a disk is damaged or ruptured, a gelatinous matter oozes from it and severe pain results from the pressure of the bones of the vertebrae on the spinal nerve roots.

As the human body passes maturity, the disks gradually shrink, causing the body to lose height. This is a complex process about which new discoveries are being made.

However, for the health of the back, careful stretching to lengthen and create space between the vertebrae is essential to allow the disks to return to a more youthful condition.

Resources

~

For Yoga Books and Videos

Rodmell Press

2550 Shattuck Ave., #18
Berkeley, CA 94704
(800) 841-3123
Fax: (510) 841-3191
e-mail: rodmellprs@aol.com

Yoga Journal's Book and Tape Source

2054 University Ave.
Berkeley, CA 94704-1082
(800) 359-YOGA (M-F, 9 A.M.-5 P.M., P.S.T.)
Fax: (510) 644-3101

For Props

Bheka Yoga Supplies

P.O. Box 147
Carlsberg, WA 98324
(800) 366-4541

Fish Crane

P.O. Box 791029
New Orleans, LA 70179
(800) 959-6116

Half Moon Yoga Props

2137 W. First Ave., Suite 2
Vancouver, B.C. V6K 1E7, Canada
(604) 731-7099

Hugger-Mugger Yoga Products

31 W. Gregson Ave.
Salt Lake City, UT 84115
(800) 473-4888

Living Arts

2434 Main St., 2nd Floor
Santa Monica, CA 90405
(800) 2-LIVING

Tools for Yoga

P.O. Box 99
Chatham, NJ 07928
(201) 966-5311

Yoga Mats

P.O. Box 885044N
San Francisco, CA 94188
(800) 720-YOGA

Yoga Pro Products

Box 7612
Ann Arbor, MI 48107
(800) 488-8414

Yoga Props

3055 23rd St.
San Francisco, CA 94110
(888) 856-YOGA

Finding a Teacher in Your Area

B.K.S., Iyengar Yoga National Association of the United States

554 Orme Circle N.E.
Atlanta, GA
(800) 889-YOGA

Provides a complete listing of certified Iyengar Yoga instructors. Visit their Web page at http://www.iyoga.com/iynaus/

International Association of Yoga Therapists

20 Sunnyside Ave., Suite A-243
Mill Valley, CA 94941
(415) 332-2478

Provides an international network and resource guide for yoga and yoga therapy.

Yoga International's Guide to Yoga Teachers and Classes

RR 1, Box 407
Honesdale, PA 18431
(800) 253-6243

National and international listings of yoga teachers, centers, certification programs and yoga associations. Updated annually as a supplement to the January/February issue of *Yoga International*. Copies available year round.

Yoga Journal's Yoga Teachers Directory

2054 University Ave., Suite 600
Berkeley, CA 94704
(800) 359-YOGA
Web site: http://www.yogajournal.com

Directory of yoga teachers in the United States, Canada and internationally. Updated annually in the July/August issue of *Yoga Journal;* also available as a special reprint. Includes listing of yoga teacher-training programs.

Resources for Conscious Aging

Omega Institute for Holistic Studies
260 Lake Drive
Rhinebeck, NY 12572-3212
(800) 944-1001

Information on Workshops with the Author

Ojai Yoga Center
P.O. Box 1258
Ojai, CA 93024
(805) 646-4673
Fax: (805) 640-8232
e-mail: sfrancina@aol.com

About Yoga in the Ojai Valley

Surrounded by majestic mountains between Los Angeles and Santa Barbara, the Ojai Valley in California is one of the most beautiful and sacred places on earth—a true Shangri-la only 30 minutes from the ocean. Your yoga vacation can include daily classes at the Ojai Yoga Center, hiking, visits to nearby mineral hotsprings and many spiritually oriented organizations, art galleries and cultural events. The Ojai Yoga Center is a fully equipped center located within easy walking distance of hotels, motels and shops. Write or call for a brochure.

Bibliography

～

Bringing home a book to read is like having the author over for a visit. I've always been an avid reader, and it is impossible to list all the books that have influenced my perspective on yoga and life. The following publications were consulted during the writing of *The New Yoga for People Over 50,* and many are quoted or cited in the text. Many more excellent books are available on all aspects of yoga, health, the stages of life, aging, conscious dying and death. I encourage you to browse through your local bookstore and read those books that speak to you.

Yoga, Health and Aging

Alberg, Maria. *The Yoga Workbook for Seniors,* Sandpoint, Idaho: Moon in the Pearl, 1993.

Beauvoir, Simone de. *The Coming of Age.* New York: G.P. Putnam's Sons, 1972.

Beeken, Jenny. *Yoga of the Heart.* Hampshire, England: White Eagle Publishing Trust, 1990.

Bell, Lorna, R.N. and Eudora Seyfer. *Gentle Yoga for People with Arthritis, Stroke Damage, Multiple Sclerosis or People in Wheelchairs.* Berkeley, Calif.: Celestial Arts, 1987.

Bender, Ruth. *Be Young and Flexible After 30, 40, 50, 60.* Avon, Conn.: Ruben Publishing, 1976.

_____. *Yoga Exercises for Every Body.* Avon, Conn.: Ruben Publishing, 1976.

Bianchi, Eugene C. *Aging as a Spiritual Journey.* New York: Crossroad Publishing Co., 1989.

Brennan, Barbara. *Hands of Light: A Guide to Healing Through the Human Energy Field.* New York: Bantam Books, 1988.

Breslow, Rachelle. *Who Said So? A Woman's Fascinating Journey of Self-Discovery and Full Recovery from Multiple Sclerosis.* Berkeley, Calif.: Celestial Arts, 1991.

Burgio, Kathryn, Ph.D. *Staying Dry: A Practical Guide to Bladder Control.* Baltimore: Johns Hopkins University Press, 1989.

Chopra, Deepak. *Ageless Body, Timeless Mind: The Quantum Alternative to Growing Old.* New York: Harmony Books, 1993.

_____. *Perfect Health: The Complete Mind/Body Guide.* New York: Harmony Books, 1991.

_____. *Quantum Healing, Exploring the Frontiers of Mind/Body Medicine.* New York: Bantam Books, 1989.

_____. *Unconditional Life.* New York: Bantam Books, 1992.

Christensen, Alice, and David Rankin. *Easy Does It Yoga for People Over 60.* Cleveland: Saraswati Studio, 1975.

Clow, Barbara H. *Liquid Light of Sex: Understanding Your Key Life Passages.* Santa Fe: Bear & Company, 1991.

Couch, Jean. *The Runner's Yoga Book.* Berkeley, Calif.: Rodmell Press, 1990.

Cousins, Norman. *The Healing Heart.* New York: Avon, 1983.

Criswell, Eleanor. *How Yoga Works: An Introduction to Somatic Yoga.* Novato, Calif.: Freeperson Press, 1987.

Delany, Sarah, and Elizabeth Delany. *Having Our Say: The Delany Sister's First 100 Years.* New York: Kodansha America, 1993.

Desikachar, T.K.V. *Patanjali's Yoga Sutras.* Madras, India: Affiliated East–West Press, 1987.

Devi, Indra, *Forever Young, Forever Healthy.* Englewood Cliffs, N.J.: Prentice Hall, 1953.

Dossey, Larry. *Beyond Illness: Discovering the Experience of Health.* Boulder, Colo.: Shambala, 1984.

_____. *Meaning and Medicine: A Doctor's Stories of Breakthrough and Healing.* New York: Bantam Books, 1992.

_____. *Recovering the Soul: A Scientific and Spiritual Search.* New York: Bantam Books, 1989.

Douillard, John D.C. *Invincible Athletics: Awakening the Athlete in Everyone.* Lancaster, Mass.: Maharishi Ayur-Veda, 1991.

Dworkis, Sam. *ExTension: A Twenty-Minute-A-Day, Yoga-Based Program to Relax, Release and Rejuvenate the Average Stressed-Out Over 35-Year-Old Body.* New York: Poseidon Press, 1994.

Dychtwald, Ken, and Joe Flower. *Age Wave: The Challenges and Opportunities of an Aging America.* New York: Bantam Books, 1990.

Erdman, Mardi. *Undercover Exercise.* Englewood Cliffs, N.J.: Prentice Hall, 1984.

Estés, Clarissa Pinkola, Ph.D. *Women Who Run With the Wolves.* New York: Ballantine Books, 1992.

Evans, William, Ph.D., and Irwin Rosenberg, M.D. *Biomarkers: The 10 Keys to Prolonging Vitality.* New York: Simon & Schuster, 1991.

Feuerstein, Georg, and Stephen Bodian. *Living Yoga: A Comprehensive Guide for Daily Life.* New York: Putnam, 1993.

Folan, Lilias. *Yoga and Your Life.* New York: Macmillan, 1981.

Friedan, Betty. *The Fountain of Age.* New York: Simon & Schuster, 1993.

Gottlieb, Bill, ed. *New Choices in Natural Healing.* Emmaus, Pa.: Rodale Press, 1995.

Greer, Germaine. *The Change: Women, Aging and Menopause.* New York: Ballantine Books, 1991.

Groves, Dawn. *Yoga for Busy People.* San Rafael, Calif.: A New World Library, 1995.

Holloman, Dona. *Centering Down.* Italy: 1981.

Iyengar, Geeta S. *Yoga, a Gem for Women.* Spokane, Wash.: Timeless Books, 1990.

Jaidar, George. *The Soul: An Owner's Manual.* New York: Paragon House, 1995.

Johns Hopkins Medical Letter, eds. *The Johns Hopkins Medical Handbook: 100 Major Medical Disorders of People over 50.* New York: Rebus, Inc., 1992.

Kabat-Zinn, Jon. *Wherever You Go, There You Are: Mindfulness Meditation in Everyday Life.* New York: Hyperion, 1994.

Kelder, Peter. *Ancient Secret of the Fountain of Youth.* Gig Harbor, Wash.: Harbor Press, 1985.

Laird, Joan. *Ageless Exercise: A Gentle Approach for the Inactive or Physically Limited.* Williamsburg, Mich.: Angelwood Press, 1994.

Lasater, Judith, Ph.D., P.T. *Relax & Renew: Restful Yoga for Stressful Times.* Berkeley, Calif.: Rodmell Press, 1995.

Lieberman, Jacob. *Light, Medicine of the Future*. Santa Fe: 1991.

Luby, Sue, and Richard Onge. *Bodysense: Hazard Free Fitness Program for Men and Women*. Winchester, Mass.: Faber & Faber, 1986.

Main, Zilpha Pallister. *Reaching Ninety My Way*. Los Angeles: Zilpha Pallister Main, 1984.

Mehta, Mira. *How to Use Yoga: A Step-by-Step Guide to the Iyengar Method of Yoga, for Relaxation, Health and Well-Being*. New York: Smithmark, 1994.

Mehta, Silva, and Mira and Shyam Mehta. *Yoga the Iyengar Way*. New York: Alfred Knopf, 1990.

Montagu, Ashley. *Growing Young*. New York: Greenwood Press, 1989.

Moyers, Bill. *Healing and the Mind*. New York: Doubleday, 1993.

Murphy, Michael. *The Future of the Body*. Los Angeles: Jeremy P. Tarcher, Inc., 1992.

Myers, Esther. *Yoga & You: Energizing and Relaxing Yoga for New and Experienced Students*. Toronto, Canada: Random House of Canada, 1996.

Nelson, John E., M.D., and Andrea Nelson, Psy.D. *Sacred Sorrows: Embracing and Transforming Depression*. New York: Tarcher/Putnam, 1996.

Noble, Vicki. *Shakti Woman*. San Francisco: Harper, 1991.

Northrup, Christiane, M.D. *Women's Bodies, Women's Wisdom*. New York: Bantam Books, 1994.

O'Brien, Paddy. *Yoga for Women*. San Francisco: HarperCollins, 1994.

Ojeda, Linda. *Menopause Without Medicine*. Claremont, Calif.: Hunter House, 1989.

Ornish, Dean, M.D. *Dr. Dean Ornish's Program for Reversing Heart Disease*. New York: Random House, 1990.

Padus, Emrika, ed. *The Women's Encyclopedia of Health & Natural Healing*. Emmaus, Pa.: Rodale Press, 1981.

Pelletier, Kenneth R. *Longevity: Fulfilling Our Biological Potential*. New York: Dell Publishing Co., 1981.

Perez-Christiaens, Noëlle. *Sparks of Divinity*. Paris: Institut de Yoga B.K.S. Iyengar, 1976.

Pilgrim, Peace. Peace Pilgrim. Santa Fe: An Ocean Tree Book, 1982. Available from Friends of Peace Pilgrim, 43480 Cedar Ave., Hemet, CA 92344.

Radha, Swami Sivananda. *Hatha Yoga: The Hidden Language*. Boston: Shambhala, 1987.

Rountree, Cathleen. *On Women Turning 50*. San Francisco: Harper, 1993.

Scaravelli, Vanda. *Awakening the Spine.* New York: HarperCollins, 1991.

Schatz, Mary Pullig, M.D. *Back Care Basics: A Doctor's Gentle Yoga Program for Back and Neck Pain Relief.* Berkeley, Calif.: Rodmell Press, 1992.

Scheller, Mary Dale. *Growing Older, Feeling Better In Body Mind & Spirit.* Palo Alto, Calif.: Bull Publishing, 1993.

Sheehy, Gail. *New Passages: Mapping Your Life Across Time.* New York: Ballantine, 1995.

_____. *Pathfinders.* New York: Bantam Books, 1981.

_____. *The Silent Passage: Menopause.* New York: Random House, 1991.

Smith, Bob. *Yoga for a New Age: A Modern Approach to Hatha Yoga.* Englewood Cliffs, N.J.: Prentice Hall, 1982.

Steinem, Gloria. *Revolution From Within: A Book of Self-Esteem.* Boston: Little, Brown & Co., 1992.

Stewart, Mary. *Yoga Over 50: The Way to Vitality, Health and Energy in the Prime of Life.* New York: Simon & Schuster, 1994.

Tobias, Maxine, and John Patrick Sullivan. *Complete Stretching.* New York: Alfred A. Knopf, 1992.

Tobias, Maxine, and Mary Stewart. *Stretch & Relax.* Tucson, Ariz.: The Body Press (HPBooks), 1985.

Ueland, Brenda. *If You Want To Write.* Saint Paul, Minn.: Graywolf Press, 1987.

Walker, Barbara G. *The Crone: Women of Age, Wisdom, and Power.* San Francisco: Harper, 1988.

_____. *The Women's Encyclopedia of Myths and Secrets.* San Francisco: Harper, 1983.

Ward, Susan Winter. *Yoga for the Young at Heart: Gentle Stretching Exercises for Seniors.* Santa Barbara, Calif.: Capra Press, 1994.

Weed, Susun S. *Menopausal Years, the Wise Woman Way: Alternative Approaches for Women 30–90.* New York: Ash Tree Publishing, 1992.

Weininger, Ben, and Eva L. Menkin. *Aging Is a Lifelong Affair.* Los Angeles: Guild of Tutors Press, 1978.

White, Timothy. *The Wellness Guide to Lifelong Fitness.* Berkeley, Calif.: University of California at Berkeley Wellness Letter, 1993.

Whiteside, Robert L. *Agile at 80.* Pukalani, Hawaii: Robert L. Whiteside, 1989.

Wood, Beatrice. *Playing Chess with the Heart: Beatrice Wood at 100.* San Francisco: Chronicle Books, 1994.

Yogananda, Paramahansa. *Autobiography of a Yogi.* Los Angeles: Self-Realization Fellowship, 1946.

Books and Publications by and About B.K.S. Iyengar

The Art of Yoga. London: Unwin Paperbacks, 1985.

Body the Shrine, Yoga Thy Light. Bombay: published by B.I. Taraporewala for Iyengar's 60th birthday, 1978 (chapter on Yoga for Women by Geeta Iyengar).

Iyengar: His Life and Work. Palo Alto, CA: Timeless Books, 1987.

Light on Pranayama. New York: Crossroad, 1981.

Light on Yoga. New York: Schocken, 1979.

Light on the Yoga Sutras of Patanjali. London: HarperCollins, 1993.

70 Glorious Years of Yogachrya B.K.S. Iyengar. Bombay: Light on Yoga Research Trust, 1990.

Tree of Yoga. Boston: Shambhala, 1989.

Use of Props (Iyengar describes the benefits of props in old age); *Yoga and Medical Science: Yoga for Overall Health* (Iyengar); *Effect of Yogasanas on Metabolism of a Cell* (Dr. Karandikar); *Asana, Pranayama and the Circulatory System; Asana, Pranayama and Coronary Tuning; Asana, Pranayama and the Nervous System* (Dr. Krishna Raman); *Symposium on Hypertension,* and other related articles cited in text.

Effect of Asanas and Pranayama on the Endocrine System, (Dr. Karandikar); *Symposium: Women's Problems, with Geeta Iyengar; Yoga and Medical Science: Yoga for Overall Health* (Iyengar).

Publications on Conscious Dying and Death

Ansley, Helen Green. *Life's Finishing School—What Now—What Next? A Ninety Year Old's View of Death and Dying a Good Death.* Sausalito, Calif.: Institute of Noetic Sciences, 1990.

Graber, Anya Foos. *Deathing: An Intelligent Alternative for the Final Moments of Life,* rev. ed. With a preface by Ramamurti S. Mishra, M.D. York Beach, Maine: Nicolas–Hays Inc., 1992.

Krishnamurti, Jiddu. *On Living and Dying.* San Francisco: Harper, 1992.

Kübler-Ross, Elisabeth. *Death: The Final Stage of Growth.* Englewood Cliffs, N.J.: Prentice Hall, 1979.

Levine, Stephen. *Healing into Life and Death.* New York: Doubleday, 1987.

Nearing, Helen. *Loving and Leaving the Good Life.* Post Mills, Vt.: Chelsea Green Publishing Co., 1992.

Ring, Kenneth. *Life at Death.* New York: Coward, McCann & Geoghegan, 1988.

Rinpoche, Sogyal. *The Tibetan Book of Living and Dying.* San Francisco: Harper, 1992.

Wilber, Ken. *Grace and Grit: Spirituality and Healing in the Life and Death of Treya Killam Wilber.* Boston: Shambhala, 1991.

Periodicals and Additional Publications

Yoga Journal:

Burke, David. "Sri Chinmoy: Athlete of the Spirit" (September/October 1983).

Carrico, Mara. "Yoga with a Chair" (May/June 1986).

Cavanaugh, Carol. "Staying Young with Yoga" (September/October 1983).

_____. "Viparita Karani: Supported Inverted Pose" (November/December 1983).

Cogozzo, Linda. "Hatha After Hip Surgery" (May/June 1985).

Farhi, Donna. "Adho Mukha Svanasana: Downward-Facing Dog" (January/February 1994).

Francina, Suza. "Nutritional Aspects of Arthritis" (November/December 1977).

Hall, Rosemary. "Seated Sun Salutation" (March/April 1986).

Iyengar, B.K.S. "The Art of Relaxation: Savasana" (September/October 1982).

Kilmuray, Arthur. "The Safe Practice of Inversions" (November/December 1983); "Yoga: A Doctor's Prescription for Asthma" (May/June 1983); "Understanding Twists" (September/October 1984); "Sarvangasana: Shoulderstand" (September/October 1990); "Urdhva Dhanurasana-Upward-Facing Bow Pose" (November/December 1992); "Sirsasana-Headstand" (July/August 1990).

Lasater, Judith, Ph.D., RPT. "The Subtle Art of Standing Well" (September/October 1985); "Supta Virasana: Lying Down Hero Pose" (March/April 1986); "Uttanasana:

Intense Stretch Pose" (March/April 1988); "Yoga and Your Heart: Interview with Dean Ornish, M.D." (September/October 1989); "Sirsasana: Headstand" (May/June 1991); "How to Relax Deeply" (May/June 1992).

Moyer, Donald. "Baddha Konasana–Bound Angle Pose" (January/February 1987); "Virasana: Hero Pose" (March/April 1989); "Adho Mukha Svanasana: Downward Facing Dog Pose" (November/December 1989); "Ardha Matsyendrasana I: Lord of the Fishes Pose" (May/June 1992).

Myers, Esther. "Awakening the Spine With Vanda Scaravelli" (June 1996).

Sander, Ellen. "Moving Through Menopause With Yoga" (February, 1996).

Schatz, Mary, M.D. "Yoga Relief for Arthritis: A Pathologist and Yoga Teacher Offers Comprehensive Guidelines for Restoring and Maintaining Joint Health" (May/June 1985; reprints available from *Yoga Journal*); "Yoga, Circulation and Imagery" (January/February 1987); "Restorative Asanas for a Healthy Immune System" (July/August 1987); "You Can Have Healthy Bones! Preventing Osteoporosis with Exercise, Diet and Yoga" (March/ April 1988); "Exercises and Yoga Poses for Those at Risk for Osteoporotic Fractures" (March/April 1988); "Yoga and Aging" (May/June 1990); "Relief for Your Aching Back" (May/June 1992).

Steiger, Ruth. "Take-It-Easy Yoga" (November/December 1987).

Thomson, Bill. "Aging with Grace" (May/June 1990).

Wakefield, Dan. "Be Old Now" (September/October 1995).

White, Ganga. " Sting on Yoga" (December 1995).

Iyengar Yoga Institute Review:

Cavanaugh, Carol. "An Interview with Dr. S.V. Karandikar" (February 1984).

_____. "Vera Sida Interview" (November 1986).

Cole, Roger, Ph.D. "Physiology of Yoga" (October 1985).

Schatz, Mary Pullig, M.D. "Stress and Relaxation—Hypertension and Yoga" (March 1984).

Transcription of the video on *"Menopause"* produced by the Institute in Pune, India. Transcript by Kay Parry, with help from Janet and Susan Robertson. Edited by Geeta Iyengar.

The Journal of the International Association of Yoga Therapists:

Arpita, Ph.D., "Physiological and Psychological Effects of Hatha Yoga: A Review of the Literature" volume 1, nos. I & II (1990).

Chandra, F.J. "Medical and Physiological Aspects of Headstand" volume 1, nos. I and II (1990). (Article from booklet series by Dr. Chandra and Ian Rawlinson.)

_____. "Yoga and the Cardiovascular System" volume 2, no. I (1991).

Dreaver, Jim. "The Ultimate Cure: Enlightenment in Daily Life", nos. I and II, (1990).

Hymes, Alan, and Phil Nuernberger, Ph.D. "Breathing Patterns in Heart Attack Patients" 2, no. I (1991). (Article from *Research Bulletin of the Himalayan International Institute,* 2, no. 2, 1980).

Martin, Donna. "Chronic Pain and Yoga Therapy" 1, nos. I and II (1990).

Lyn, Brian. "Reflex (psychophysical yoga)" 1, nos. I and II (1990).

Mayer, Tania. "The Dance of Healing: Multiple Sclerosis and Yoga Therapy" 1, nos. I and II (1990).

Miller, Richard. "The Psychophysiology of Respiration: Eastern and Western Perspectives" 2, no. I (1991). (Article from booklet series published by Cambridge Yoga Publications.)

Miscellaneous Publications

Adolph, Jonathan. "The Wisdom Years: Five Reasons to Look Forward to Old Age." *New Age Journal,* (March/April 1992).

Blakeney, Laurie, Rose Richardson, Sue Salaniuk, and Toni Fuhrman. "Interview with B.K.S. Iyengar." Yoga '93 conference publication.

Clark, Etta. "Growing Old Is Not for Sissies." *The Sun* 196 (1992).

Dunn, Mary. "In Praise of Props: Utilizing the Mundane to Effect the Miraculous." Yoga '87 conference publication.

Eskenazi, Kay and Ruth Steiger. "Backbending Bench Usage Guide," "Eyesbag Usage Guide," "Halasana Bench Usage Guide," "Headstander Usage Guide," "Pelvic Swing Usage Guide, Pranayama Bolster Usage Guide, Wall Ropes Usage Guide." These booklets are highly recommended and may be purchased through Yoga Props. Please see address, page 268.

Hendrix, Paula. "Confessions of a Nursing Home Worker" and "Natural Dying." *In Context* no. 31 (1992).

Johns Hopkins White Papers, 1993: Arthritis, Coronary Heart Disease, Hypertension.

Schatz, Mary Pullig, M.D. "Minimizing Pain: The Principles of Therapeutic Yoga." Yoga '87 conference publication.

Weil, Andrew. "High Blood Pressure: Controlling Hypertension Without Drugs". *East-West Journal* (May/June 1992).

Permissions *(Continued from page iv)*

Photographs on pages 89, 91, 92, 95, 98, 164, and 213 reprinted with permission of Judi Flannery Lukas. ©1992 Judi Flannery Lukas.

Photograph on page 247 reprinted with permission of Cynthia MacAdams. ©1992 Cynthia MacAdams.

Photograph on page 261 reprinted with permission of Dot Coykendal. ©1993 Dot Coykendal.

Photograph on page 263 reprinted with permission of Jody Kasch. ©1993 Jody Kasch.

Photograph on page 7 reprinted with permission of Rob Howard. ©1990 Rob Howard.

Quotes from *Awakening the Spine* by Vanda Scaravelli. ©1991 by Vanda Scaravelli. Reprinted with permission of HarperCollins Publishers, Inc.

The Tree of Yoga, pp. 31-34. From *The Tree of Yoga,* by B. K. S. Iyengar. ©1988 by B. K. S. Iyengar. Reprinted by arrangement with Shambhala Publications, Inc., P.O. Box 308, Boston, MA, 02117.

Back Care Basics: A Doctor's Gentle Yoga Program for Back and Neck Pain Relief, by Mary Pullig Schatz, M.D. ©1992 by Mary Pullig Schatz, M.D. Reprinted with permission of Rodmell Press, Berkeley, CA.

Healing and the Mind. Excerpt published with permission by Doubleday, a division of Bantam Doubleday Dell Publishing Group. ©1993 by Bill Moyers.

Hatha Yoga: The Hidden Language. Excerpt, pp. 259-260, reprinted with permission of Timeless Books, Spokane, WA, by Swami Sivananda Radha. ©1987 by Swami Sivananda Radha.

Biomarkers. Reprinted with permission of Simon & Schuster, from BIOMARKERS by William Evans, Ph.D., and Irwin H. Rosenberg, M.D. ©1991 by Dr. Irwin H. Rosenberg, Dr. William J. Evans, and Jacqueline Thompson.

Bodysense: The Hazard-Free Fitness Program for Men and Women, by Sue Luby, Faber & Faber, Inc., Winchester, MA. Excerpt reprinted by permission of Sue Luby. ©1986 by Sue Luby.

Yoga: A Gem for Women, p. 52. Excerpt reprinted with permission by Timeless Books, Spokane, WA, ©1990 by Geeta S. Iyengar.

Gentle Yoga, page 3. Excerpted from *Gentle Yoga,* ©1982, 1987 by Lorna Bell, R.N., and Eudora Seyfer, with permission by Celestial Arts, P.O. Box 7327, Berkeley, CA 94707.

Complete Stretching. Excerpt from *Complete Stretching,* by Maxine Tobias and John Patrick Sullivan, published with permission by Random House, Inc., New York, NY, 1992.

Revolution from Within. Excerpt from *Revolution from Within,* by Gloria Steinem, published with permission by Little Brown and Company Publishers, Boston, MA, 1992.

Perfect Health. Excerpt from *Perfect Health* by Deepak Chopra, M.D., published with permission of Harmony Books, a division of Crown Publisher, New York, NY, 1991.

Relax & Renew: Restful Yoga for Stressful Times, by Judith Lasater, Ph.D., P.T. ©1995 by Judith Lasater, Ph.D., P.T. Reprinted with permission of Rodmell Press, Berkeley, CA.

About the Author

～

Suza Francina is a certified Iyengar Yoga instructor with more than 20 years of experience in the field of yoga and exercise therapy. Her interest in teaching older people began many years ago while she worked as a home health-care provider for elderly and convalescing people. Her relationship with her clients extended through the last years of their lives. Francina's articles on health and aging have appeared in *Prevention, Yoga Journal, Women's Health Care—A Guide to Alternatives, The Holistic Health Handbook, American Yoga* and other publications. Her first book, a completely different *Yoga for People Over 50*, was published in 1977.

Born in The Hague, Holland, Suza Francina has lived in Ojai, California for over 40 years. She is director of the Ojai Yoga Center where she specializes in classes and workshops for people over 50. In addition to teaching yoga, Francina has a deep interest in spiritual politics—a new emerging paradigm that recognizes the sacred interconnection of all life. She is a spokesperson for sustainable lifestyles, serves on the Ojai City Council and writes extensively on health and environmental issues.

Index of Poses

~

AUTHOR'S NOTE: *This index does not list the more advanced postures demonstrated in this book. These are best learned under the guidance of a yoga teacher.*

285